THE DIET TRAP
SOLUTION

Also by Judith S. Beck PhD

The Beck Diet Solution: Train Your Brain to Think Like a Thin Person

The Beck Diet Solution: Weight Loss Workbook

The Complete Beck Diet for Life

Cognitive Behavior Therapy: Basics and Beyond (2nd edition)

Cognitive Therapy for Challenging Problems: What to Do When the Basics Don't Work

The Oxford Textbook of Psychotherapy

Cognitive Therapy of Personality Disorders

THE DIET TRAP SOLUTION

Train Your Brain to Lose Weight and Keep It Off for Good

JUDITH S. BECK PhD
& DEBORAH BECK BUSIS

HAY HOUSE

Carlsbad, California • New York City • London • Sydney
Johannesburg • Vancouver • Hong Kong • New Delhi

First published and distributed in the United Kingdom by:
Hay House UK Ltd, Astley House, 33 Notting Hill Gate, London W11 3JQ
Tel: +44 (0)20 3675 2450; Fax: +44 (0)20 3675 2451; www.hayhouse.co.uk

First published and distributed in the United States of America by:
HarperOne, 195 Broadway, New York, NY 10007
www.harpercollins.com

Published and distributed in the Republic of South Africa by:
Hay House SA (Pty) Ltd, PO Box 990, Witkoppen 2068
info@hayhouse.co.za

Published and distributed in India by:
Hay House Publishers India, Muskaan Complex, Plot No.3, B-2,
Vasant Kunj, New Delhi 110 070
Tel: (91) 11 4176 1620; Fax: (91) 11 4176 1630; www.hayhouse.co.in

A catalogue record for this book is available from the British Library.

ISBN: 978-1-78180-589-3

Designed by Terry McGrath

Printed and bound in Great Britain by TJ International Ltd, Padstow, Cornwall

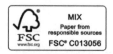

Contents

PART ONE

Escape Your Diet Traps

Chapter 1

Are You Trapped?

Diet books, diet plans, diet programs. They all want you to believe they have the magic formula. Eat what they say, and losing weight will be easy and quick.

If that's true, why are two-thirds of Americans overweight? Why do most people who lose weight gain it back? And not just once but over and over again?

We're going to tell you the truth: Losing weight can be easy at first, but continuing to lose weight after the first few weeks or months, and then keeping off the weight you lose, can be very difficult. That is, unless you've learned how to identify the problems—the traps—that you're certain to encounter, and figured out how to develop escape plans for each one.

We all face plenty of traps. Stress, family problems, and food pushers are some of the negatives of life. But there are also vacations, celebrations, holidays—the positives of life. All these situations can create traps when your goal is to lose weight.

Without special plans to address these real-life situations, keeping weight off can be a constant and draining battle, and studies show that most people fail in the long run. Why? Because having an eating plan is not enough. Using an app or a website isn't enough. Even having someone else prepare your food and deliver it to your doorstep isn't enough.

You need something more—something you'll never be able to whip up in a blender or buy in a store. You need to learn *how* to lose weight. *How* to motivate yourself every day. *How* to change sabotaging thinking ("It's okay to eat the last piece of birthday cake because otherwise it will just go to waste!"). *How* to get yourself back on track whenever you make a mistake.

In this book, you will learn how to create your own personal escape plans to help you get out of your stickiest traps. You'll acquire the tools you need to prevent or escape from the traps all around you—the traps you create, traps that other people create, traps that life circumstances create, and even certain universal traps that we all encounter.

To be successful, you *do* need an eating plan. But your success will not be determined exclusively by protein or carbs or fiber. You will experience success when you learn *how* to stick to your plan *even when you don't feel like it*—when you're stressed or upset, when people push food on you, when you're eating out at your favorite restaurant, even when you're traveling, attending a special event, or celebrating your birthday. The escape plans you create will contain the solutions you need when temptation strikes. They will detail exactly what you need to say to yourself and what strategies you need to use when a trap threatens to throw you off course.

This approach has helped thousands of dieters stick to their plans and lose weight, even when confronted with challenge after challenge. Take Jessica, for example. Jessica came to see me after almost fifteen years of struggling with her weight. Since college, she had gained and lost the same forty pounds several times. Now struggling to balance her personal health goals with her hectic career as an HR manager, Jessica felt disheartened, ready to give up.

Jessica knew all about sound nutrition, and she could recite the pros and cons of just about every popular weight-loss program. She knew the facts cold—but those facts were no help when she was upset. She desperately wanted to learn how to stop eating when she wasn't hungry, especially when she needed to soothe herself. She knew her favorite chocolate-covered pretzels, caramel popcorn, and mini-doughnuts weren't healthy, but that was what she craved when she had a fight with her partner or was anxious about missing a deadline at work.

"I do okay a lot of the time," she told me, "but when I'm upset, I go right for the sweets. I know I shouldn't. I know every time I do, it sets me back." She sighed. "I can't help it. I'm just so weak. Food is the only thing that calms me down."

Jessica's difficulties are a prime example of the emotional eating trap. She didn't realize that her biggest challenge wasn't feeling distressed; it was what she was *telling herself* about feeling distressed. She had convinced herself that she simply couldn't cope without eating.

No wonder she was trapped. She had completely bought into the idea that food was the only solution when she was upset. An important aspect of Jessica's ultimate success in losing weight was proving to herself that this simply wasn't true. Being human, Jessica will always experience negative emotions. She just had to learn how to cope with them differently.

Here's the cold, hard truth: the headaches of life don't care that you want to lose weight. Difficulties with work, with relationships, with finances or health—these things never go away. No matter how unjust it may feel, life will never stop presenting you with challenging moments and situations—and in each of those moments and situations, temptations to eat. Those temptations are easier to resist when you're feeling strong and committed. But when you feel weak or impulsive, they can seem unavoidable, inescapable, completely unfair.

They can feel like traps—with a capital *T*.

How These Things Usually Go

If you've tried to lose weight before, chances are your experience went something like this:

❶ **You find a diet plan that implies you won't need willpower and discipline.** You believe the hype that the plan will "automatically" make dieting (and then maintenance) painless. "Just follow the plan and the pounds will melt off," they promise. And you feel certain: Yes. Finally. This is *the One*.

❷ **You want to believe in the magic.** (Who doesn't?) You buy into the fantasy that dieting will be easy. You believe that this new diet will eliminate your hunger so you can lose all the weight you want in a short time.

❸ **With your plan in hand, you . . . don't start right away.** Instead, you have one last blowout, eating everything you want in whatever quantity you want. You think, "This is my last chance—I'm going to enjoy it!" You may even put on a few extra pounds as you overeat pasta, pizza, cupcakes, french fries, chips, cookies—foods that aren't on your new diet plan. You tell yourself that it doesn't matter because "I'll start my diet on Monday!"

❹ **You stock up on whatever magical formula your plan prescribes.** Maybe it's grapefruit or quinoa, maybe certain brands of low-fat frozen meals or Greek yogurt. Maybe you stuff your veggie drawer until it's overflowing with kale and beets. You toss the chocolate and the ice cream. You start to measure your food, eat at prescribed intervals, drink eight glasses of water, and step up your exercise. Like a soldier on a mission, you're focused and determined. You've got this.

❺ **And—here's the kicker—it works! Temporarily.** You lose a lot of weight (okay, true, most of it is water weight) the first week, and you feel excited and optimistic. You find it pretty easy because your motivation is high. (Why else would you be starting a diet right now?) The pounds seem to melt away. No sweat!

❻ **You expect that every week will go as smoothly as the first few.** You think, "At this rate, I'm sure to get to my goal in no time." And then you fool yourself into thinking you'll be able to stop dieting and go back to eating your favorite foods, and the pounds will stay off. Finally. You think you've really figured it out this time.

❼ **But then . . .** your best friend or your mother or your daughter-in-law makes a special dinner for the two of you. Caesar salad, lasagna, and homemade garlic bread with lots of butter. And—how nice!—she made brownies with crushed nuts, just the way you like them.

Well, you might reason, just this once. She worked so hard. You really want her to know how touched you are. You'll just eat part of the salad. But it tastes so good! And you don't want to hurt her feelings by not finishing it. She serves you a really big portion of lasagna. It'll be okay. Just this once. The bread—hard to stop at just one piece. And you can't pass up the brownies.

Oh well, this is a special occasion. You can start again tomorrow.

But tomorrow you give yourself one more day of eating whatever you feel like. And maybe another day after that, and another day after that. . . .

No wonder you fell off the wagon. You never really learned how to handle this type of situation. No one ever taught you how to prepare yourself for tempting situations, how to keep your eye on your long-term goal, or how to stick to your plan even when you don't feel like it. It isn't your fault. You just didn't know how.

The Traps Are Set and Waiting

Even if dieting starts out easy, the moment inevitably comes when it shifts into hard work. Your willpower, which seemed strong at the beginning, eventually starts to flag. The chocolate fudge ice cream tucked way back in the freezer begins loudly calling your name. The doughnuts at work make your mouth water. You feel resentful of everything your friends and family are eating. You are annoyed by how unfair it is that your coworkers eat pepperoni pizza or smothered burritos for lunch and you can't. (Or at least not in the quantity they do.)

Everyone faces these traps—situations in which you are tempted to eat or drink in a way that you'll later regret. The circumstances that blind you for those seconds between "I really *shouldn't* eat that" and "Darn it, I really *shouldn't have* eaten that." Your own particular vulnerabilities. Your dieting Achilles's heels.

Well, no more. We are here to tell you that there is a solution. Your traps don't have to ensnare you any longer. You can learn precisely what to do to avoid your traps—and if you fall into one, how to get out immediately and put yourself back on track.

How to successfully lose weight isn't intuitively obvious—but the skills you need can be learned. Like Jessica, you'll need to craft your own personal escape plans, based on understanding why you make particular mistakes, so you'll know exactly what to do and what to say to yourself the next time you face a challenging situation.

For example, to overcome her emotional eating trap, Jessica needed to question the idea that the only way she could calm down was by eating. She was able to recall a number of times when she experienced negative emotions, even high levels of emotion, but was able to calm down without food. With her changed thinking, she was able to do some problem solving, opening her mind to other activities she could do when she was distressed. She discovered she really *could* feel soothed by a nice, hot soak in the tub for fifteen minutes with *People* magazine. And if a bath didn't do the trick, she had a list of other activities to try, none of which were followed by guilt and recrimination—or weight gain.

But identifying alternative behaviors wasn't enough. Jessica needed to learn skills to *motivate* herself to try these new behaviors. And she needed a system to remind herself, every time, that she didn't need food to calm down. That she could just accept her negative emotions without trying to change them. Or that she could refocus her attention. In short, that she absolutely *could* cope without eating. Jessica's escape plan helped change her whole orientation toward food and distress.

Once Jessica learned that she didn't need food to cope, she evened out her eating. She lost twenty pounds without much difficulty. How did she do it? With a reasonable eating and exercise program combined with an escape plan designed specifically to address her difficulties. For the first time she could remember, Jessica felt in control of her craving for sweets, even during times of strong emotion. It wasn't that the cravings never occurred; rather she knew exactly how to handle them. She felt confident that she would be able to use the techniques in *The Diet Trap Solution* to continue losing weight and then keep it off. She felt like a changed person.

As you practice the strategies in these pages, you will become more and more skilled. You'll see your own traps more clearly and be able to avoid them or overcome them more easily. Eventually, your new ways of thinking and eating will become second nature.

The Beck Team Approach

We (Judith Beck, Ph.D., and Deborah Beck Busis, LCSW, my daughter, coauthor, and diet program coordinator at the Beck Institute for Cognitive Behavior Therapy in Philadelphia) developed a program for our diet clients over the course of many years. My first book, *The Beck Diet Solu-*

tion: Train Your Brain to Think Like a Thin Person, and a workbook were based on this program. The book didn't include a diet; instead it taught dieters a series of skills to lose weight, many of which you'll read about in the next chapter.

Since that book's release, we've been blown away by the success of thousands of dieters who have followed our program. We've gotten feedback from readers on almost every continent, as the book has been translated into twenty languages. We've heard from men and women, people of all ages, socioeconomic groups, and ethnic backgrounds. They have e-mailed us, tweeted us, written posts on Facebook, or participated in our workshops or in online support groups on various websites. Through our interactions with them, we began to realize that while the book was helpful, many of these dieters needed more specific help and suggestions to deal with everyday challenges that kept tripping them up. To achieve full success, they needed to learn how to work their way through challenges and view traps as opportunities for positive change. Please note, our books are designed for dieters. People with eating disorders need a fuller cognitive behavioral approach.

Through our work with these dieters and patients over the past thirty years, we've realized that sometimes you don't see a trap until you're standing in the middle of it. Sometimes the trap is so long standing that it feels impossible to evade. But regardless of how trapped you feel, there are always solutions. Remembering to stop, refocus on your goal, and use the strategies you've learned is a reflex that can be developed. As with every other new skill or habit, the secret is *practice, practice, practice.*

We are not going to mislead you. Losing weight will never be effortless. Anyone who tells you otherwise is selling you a bill of goods. Losing weight takes determination and endurance. But once you learn to escape your traps, dieting generally becomes progressively easier, with only intermittent occasions when things get more difficult.

Most importantly, *The Diet Trap Solution* will help you respond to sabotaging thinking that makes dieting hard. You'll learn how to anticipate traps, change your sabotaging thoughts, marshal your problem-solving abilities, and develop escape plans so you become your own best ally. And you'll learn how to recover right away if you do get caught in a trap. No more waiting until tomorrow to start over. Learning to recognize and overcome diet traps is the only way you will ever win the weight-loss battle.

The Power of Your Mind

One of the most common misconceptions about weight loss is that, to succeed, you just have to focus on *what you eat.*

Not true. An equally decisive factor in successful weight loss is changing *what you think.* To get yourself to consistently *eat* differently, you must learn to *think* differently.

You may not even be aware, or fully aware, of how your thinking influences how you eat. For example, maybe you've had thoughts like these:

- "It's okay to have extra pizza because I had a bad day."

- "It's unfair that I can't eat like everyone else."

- "I know I shouldn't eat this whole sub sandwich, but I can't resist."

If you've had these kinds of thoughts, chances are you didn't know how to counter them. You probably took them at face value, as simple truths—and ended up eating more than you had planned. Then you may have had another sabotaging thought:

- "I've already messed up, so I might as well eat whatever I want for the rest of the day and start again tomorrow."

If you did continue on that path, you may also have had another kind of sabotaging thought, one that undermines your sense of self-control:

- "I'm so weak."

- "I can't believe I cheated on my diet!"

- "I did it again. I'll never be able to lose weight."

Sound familiar? This kind of thinking is Kryptonite for your self-confidence. When these thoughts go unanswered, they set you up for failure. They demoralize you and make it all the more difficult to get back on track. They also erode your willpower, so you continue to make one eating mistake after another.

The only way to lose weight and keep it off for the long term is to learn how to challenge these unhelpful ideas. Because really, that's all they are: ideas. Not truths. When these unhelpful thoughts arise, you need a powerful way to respond, to remind yourself *why* you want to stick to your plan and exactly how you can do it, no matter what trap you are circling at the time.

Learning to identify—and respond effectively to—unhelpful, unrealistic thinking and to develop concrete solutions to problems are key features of Cognitive Behavior Therapy, also known as CBT. (*Cognition* is another word for "thinking.") CBT is a form of talk therapy that has been demonstrated in over a thousand clinical trials to be effective for a wide range of psychological and behavioral problems. Aaron T. Beck, MD (our father and grandfather, respectively), is known throughout the world for developing this modality of treatment in the 1960s and refining it ever since.

In recent times, CBT has become the standard of care among many psychologists who help people control their eating. In a survey of over 1,300 licensed psychologists conducted by the American Psychological Association in conjunction with *Consumer Reports*,[1] seven of ten psychologists selected the techniques of CBT as among the most effective strategies they use with patients who are facing diet and weight-loss challenges. CBT has been shown to help everyone from people with just a few pounds to lose all the way to those who struggle with chronic obesity and binge-eating disorder.[2]

We have used CBT with great success in our Philadelphia clinic. Both of us travel the world teaching CBT for weight loss and maintenance to health and mental health professionals, to doctors and nurses, and to coaches, trainers, and dietitians. We consult with researchers and weight-loss programs and write about dieting and maintenance for a variety of media. Over and over again, professionals and consumers tell us, "What you say makes so much sense. Why doesn't every weight-loss program include CBT?" We have been so gratified to see this approach literally change lives.

The heart of CBT is awareness and change. CBT teaches you how to identify thoughts and feelings that trigger unhelpful behavior. By becoming more aware of your sabotaging thinking, you can slow down and question your assumptions. This moment of conscious reflection gives you the chance to make a different choice. Instead of immediately reaching for an extra slice of pizza, you learn how to stop and make a different decision.

Imagine what might happen the next time you see a plate of delicious cookies you hadn't planned to eat. In the past, you might have simply accepted sabotaging thoughts like these:

- "I can't resist."

- "It's okay if I only have one."

- "Just this one time won't matter. I'll make up for it later."

But imagine what could happen if you had prepared for this moment by regularly and repeatedly reading these "reminder cards" to change your thinking:

> I'm absolutely not eating this because it's unplanned extra food. If I do give in, I'll get a few moments of pleasure but then feel bad afterward—for so much longer. And I'll put myself at risk for eating off plan for the rest of the day. It's not worth it!

> Since I want to lose weight for good, I have to take every opportunity to resist unplanned food. In a few minutes, I'm going to feel so proud of myself for not giving in.

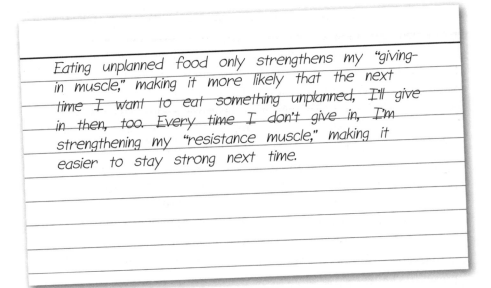

Eating unplanned food only strengthens my "giving-in muscle," making it more likely that the next time I want to eat something unplanned, I'll give in then, too. Every time I don't give in, I'm strengthening my "resistance muscle," making it easier to stay strong next time.

Once you learn how to firmly respond to your sabotaging thinking, losing weight will become progressively easier. You'll remember to say to yourself, "Eating this extra food *matters*! Every time matters!" And you'll build up your confidence that you can resist traps and succeed in following your plan. By changing how you think, you can also change how you feel and what you do. You have the power to change your thoughts—and changing those thoughts truly can change your life.

Change Your Thoughts, Change Your Brain

Even if you've been thinking in unhelpful ways for many years, you will practice your new ways of thinking and behaving until they become almost automatic. The approach is straightforward and powerful.

Recent research in neuroscience has demonstrated the changes that CBT brings about in your brain. When you think in a certain way for a long time, your brain becomes more and more efficient at thinking that way. You can drive your car, catch the subway or bus, or brush your teeth practically on autopilot, right? You may not even be aware of the automatic thoughts preceding behaviors that seem to just happen without any intentional action from you.

The reason these activities *seem* automatic is that you have trained your brain: you have allowed these thoughts and behaviors to entrench themselves over many years of doing or thinking the same thing. You no longer have to consciously think about what to do, in which order, when you slide behind the driver's seat in your car. The alternatives have been selectively "pruned out" of your brain: their neural pathways withered away from disuse. Your current patterns of thinking and behavior got woven into the networks in your brain, where they repeat over and over and over.

But this is key: if you wanted to, you *could* change these thoughts and behaviors at any time. You could look in your rearview mirror only *after* you pulled the car out into the street. You could turn on your turn signal only after you had made a turn. You could speed up when you approach a red light—or slam on the brakes as you approach a green. Those choices *are* possible. We have power of choice, and therefore we also have the power to change.

While scientists once believed our brains to be static and immutable past a certain age, we know now that our brains are "plastic"—they continue to learn from the moment we're born, and they never stop changing. CBT provides a system for changing your thinking, deliberately and methodically, so you can change your behavior.

Now, it won't happen overnight. You may have had years (or decades) of giving in to sabotaging thoughts. But practicing new ways of thinking—every day—will help you change your responses to the traps you'll encounter. In fact, studies have shown that CBT can actually produce physical changes in your brain.

Using sophisticated magnetic resonance imaging (MRI) equipment, researchers have traced changes in the brains of people who received CBT for chronic pain and entrenched addictions, severe phobias, obsessive-compulsive disorder, and major depression.[3] Using some of the techniques we share in this book, these patients were able to harness the power of their minds to change their mood and behavior and overcome serious problems, in some cases more effectively than with medication—and without side effects. Decades of research demonstrate it really works.

By using these techniques over and over, by learning how to challenge your sabotaging thoughts and consciously choose an alternate behavior, not only do you change your habits but you can also change your brain structure. You *can* change the way you think. You *can* succeed at weight loss.

How a Trap Forms

Eating is obviously necessary to sustain life. We are driven to eat when we're hungry. But we also eat for other reasons: to satisfy a craving, to experience pleasure, to be social, to soothe, to celebrate, to suppress negative emotions, to cope with stress. Many of our cultural and religious traditions and holidays include food and drink. Birthday cakes, happy hour, holiday dinners—almost every social gathering incorporates food or drink, and the sustenance and pleasure that come from food can bring people together in a positive shared experience. Much like another pleasurable biological function—procreation!—we are hardwired on an evolutionary level to enjoy eating for a simple reason: it keeps the human race alive.

But the attitude that you should be able to eat whatever you want, whenever you want, is problematic. You may develop unhelpful eating patterns that can be difficult to change. You know intellectually that you'd be much better off eating more healthily, but at the moment of temptation, your sabotaging thinking leads you straight into a trap.

Once you learn to use the strategies of CBT, you'll be able to make choices, in the moment, that move you toward your goal of lasting weight loss. You will start to resist traps. Even when you do fall into a trap, you'll have the skills to get yourself out.

Your mind is immensely powerful. Your brain has the ability to change and keep changing.

Our Many and Varied Traps

We all encounter traps. Anyone who has struggled with losing weight has fallen into traps. Each one contains a number of sabotaging thoughts. Do some of these statements ring a bell with you?

Emotional eating traps: "If I'm upset, I deserve to eat."

Stress traps: "I'm too busy and overwhelmed to keep on dieting."

Food pusher traps: "I can't disappoint people by turning down food they're offering me."

Family traps: "I shouldn't ask my family to make changes just because I want to lose weight."

Travel and eating out traps: "It's okay to indulge when I'm away."

Holiday traps: "It's a special time. I should be able to eat whatever I want."

Psychological traps: "I have no willpower. I just can't resist."

Getting off track traps: "I've already blown it for the day. I might as well keep eating and get back on track tomorrow."

Everyone has his or her personal assortment of diet traps. Maybe every time you visit your family, you find yourself overindulging. Maybe you munch on crunchy snacks or candy that you hadn't planned to eat during stressful times at work. Maybe you're disciplined during the week but can't resist overindulging in those wings and nachos at happy hour on Friday. (You know you shouldn't, but just the thought of them pulls you through the last two hours of the workweek.)

You may have thought all along that it was *a situation* itself that drove you to eat more than you'd planned. Or perhaps you believed that eating was automatic ("I don't know what happened. Suddenly the bag of chips was empty!"). But unlike bodily functions like the beating of your heart, eating is not automatic. There's no direct unbreakable connection between a situation and an eating behavior. Eating is always influenced by what you think. For example:

Situation: You are offered an extra piece of cake at a birthday party.

Sabotaging thought: "It's okay to eat it. I'll make up for it later."

Behavior: You eat the cake. And later feel bad that you did.

A different outcome occurs, however, once you learn to pause and remember that you can escape this trap with a different response.

Same trigger: You are offered an extra piece of cake.

Same sabotaging thought: "It's okay to eat it. I'll make up for it later."

Response: [this time you pause, reflect on your goals, and say to yourself] "No, I'm definitely not going to eat this. If I do, I'll get a few moments of pleasure, but I'll feel mad at myself later. Besides, I won't enjoy it that much, because I'll feel guilty about eating it. Making exceptions has always gotten me into trouble in the past. It's not worth it."

Behavior: This time, you pass up the extra cake. And feel proud of yourself.

Those critical few seconds of pause and response make all the difference. *The Diet Trap Solution* teaches you to anticipate high-risk situations, predict what your sabotaging thinking will be, and rehearse helpful responses before difficult circumstances arise.

The multipart quiz starting on page 19 will help you figure out which traps are most challenging for you. Then you'll begin to master the foundation strategies that will be crucial to overcoming the traps that plague you. Finally, you'll create personalized escape plans, integrating the foundation strategies with specific strategies designed for each trap. As you go along, you'll discover that you can use this integrated approach not only to help you lose weight but also to achieve your goals in other challenging situations.

How You Can Learn to Escape Traps

We describe eight types of traps in this book. You'll meet a number of dieters (real-life clients but with names and some personal details changed) encountering their own traps. You'll see how sabotaging thinking got them in trouble, how they fell into traps, and what they did and said to themselves to avoid these traps. You'll learn key cognitive and behavioral skills that will help you motivate yourself every day, challenge the inner voice that tries to sabotage your efforts, and get back on track when you falter. You'll learn a step-by-step process to combine the strategies that are most effective for you, so you can start laying down those new neural pathways. Through stories, examples, and specific tips, you'll learn important skills:

Cognitive strategies to help you change your mind-set

Motivational strategies that remind you why sticking to your plan is worthwhile, no matter the circumstances

Psychological strategies to help you manage issues such as feeling discouraged, deprived, burdened, unmotivated, or apathetic

Behavioral strategies to help you establish new habits

Problem-solving strategies to help you troubleshoot everyday challenges

In the final section of each trap chapter, you will identify the situations that are most challenging for you and craft an escape plan for each. You'll zero in on your own sabotaging thoughts and behaviors. You'll apply the strategies you've learned to address unhelpful self-talk, solve real-life problems, discipline yourself consistently, implement behavioral changes, and manage the psychological issues that throw you off track. You will *finally* be able to make changes in your eating that you can maintain for the long run.

Cognitive Behavior Therapy really is the missing link in your weight-loss journey. Using this approach, you will learn how to get out of your own way and reap the benefits of losing weight:

Being leaner and healthier

Having more energy

Increasing your self-confidence

Feeling in control and not at the mercy of food

Feeling more attractive

Providing a healthy role model for your kids

Enjoying shopping for clothes

Being more confident at work and in social situations

And many, many other benefits, some of which you may not even recognize until later

You don't need fancy equipment. You don't need to pay high membership fees or order special meals. You can follow whatever healthy, maintainable diet you want; we simply teach you to stay on it.

QUIZ: What Are Your Biggest Traps?

In the pages of this book, you will find the eight traps that tend to challenge dieters most. Almost every dieter who struggles to lose weight or keep it off struggles with these traps. Once you figure out which traps catch you most often, you can create escape plans so you'll know exactly what to do when you are most vulnerable.

Take this quiz to identify your own traps. After you are consistently using each foundation strategy from chapter 2 every day, turn to the chapters that correspond to your traps to craft a personalized program targeted to your specific issues.

SCORING:

For every "Not at all likely," give yourself 0 points.
For every "Slightly likely," give yourself 1 point.
For every "Moderately likely," give yourself 2 points.
For every "Very likely," give yourself 3 points.

Any trap in which you score 5 or above is an issue for you; you may need to read and reread those chapters to help you internalize those strategies. But also make sure to read any chapter for which you answered "Moderately likely," with special attention on those for which you answered "Very likely."

1. How likely are you to use food to relax after a stressful day?

  ☐ Not at all likely   ☐ Slightly likely   ☐ Moderately likely   ☐ Very likely

2. How likely are you to turn to fast food or less-healthy, easy-access food options when you're stressed?

☐ Not at all likely   ☐ Slightly likely   ☐ Moderately likely   ☐ Very likely

3. How likely are you to say to yourself, "I am too busy to diet right now"?

☐ Not at all likely   ☐ Slightly likely   ☐ Moderately likely   ☐ Very likely

STRESS TOTAL _____

4. How likely are you to turn to food when you're upset?

☐ Not at all likely   ☐ Slightly likely   ☐ Moderately likely   ☐ Very likely

5. How likely are you to eat more than you should when you're tired, bored, or procrastinating?

☐ Not at all likely   ☐ Slightly likely   ☐ Moderately likely   ☐ Very likely

6. How likely are you to think, "Eating is the only thing that helps me feel better" or "If I'm upset I deserve to eat"?

☐ Not at all likely   ☐ Slightly likely   ☐ Moderately likely   ☐ Very likely

EMOTIONAL EATING TOTAL _____

7. How likely are you to say to yourself, "I have to eat it; I don't want to be rude."

☐ Not at all likely   ☐ Slightly likely   ☐ Moderately likely   ☐ Very likely

8. How likely are you to cave to peer pressure when people urge you to drink or eat more than you think you should?

☐ Not at all likely   ☐ Slightly likely   ☐ Moderately likely   ☐ Very likely

9. How likely are you to feel unentitled to turn down food that isn't on your eating plan?

☐ Not at all likely   ☐ Slightly likely   ☐ Moderately likely   ☐ Very likely

FOOD PUSHERS TOTAL _____

10. How likely are you to overeat when your family upsets you?

☐ Not at all likely   ☐ Slightly likely   ☐ Moderately likely   ☐ Very likely

11. How likely are you to go off plan during family meals or gatherings?

☐ Not at all likely   ☐ Slightly likely   ☐ Moderately likely   ☐ Very likely

12. How likely are you to keep your family happy instead of doing what you need to do to lose weight (e.g., keeping "high-risk" foods in the house, accommodating their eating schedule, putting away leftovers yourself)?

☐ Not at all likely   ☐ Slightly likely   ☐ Moderately likely   ☐ Very likely

FAMILY PROBLEMS TOTAL _____

13. How likely are you to go to a restaurant or an event without a plan for what you're going to eat?

☐ Not at all likely   ☐ Slightly likely   ☐ Moderately likely   ☐ Very likely

14. How likely are you to say, "All diets are off!" while on vacation?

☐ Not at all likely   ☐ Slightly likely   ☐ Moderately likely   ☐ Very likely

15. How likely are you to overindulge when you're out socially?

☐ Not at all likely   ☐ Slightly likely   ☐ Moderately likely   ☐ Very likely

TRAVEL AND EATING OUT TOTAL _____

16. How likely are you to see holiday parties as a "diet-free zone"?

☐ Not at all likely   ☐ Slightly likely   ☐ Moderately likely   ☐ Very likely

17. How likely are you to say to yourself, "I'll start watching my eating once the holidays are over"?

☐ Not at all likely   ☐ Slightly likely   ☐ Moderately likely   ☐ Very likely

18. How likely are you to gain more than one or two pounds during the holiday season?

☐ Not at all likely   ☐ Slightly likely   ☐ Moderately likely   ☐ Very likely

HOLIDAYS TOTAL _____

19. How likely are you to feel discouraged or burdened by dieting?

☐ Not at all likely   ☐ Slightly likely   ☐ Moderately likely   ☐ Very likely

20. How likely are you to feel a sense of deprivation or unfairness when you see what other people are eating?

☐ Not at all likely   ☐ Slightly likely   ☐ Moderately likely   ☐ Very likely

21. How likely are you to say to yourself, "No wonder I can't lose weight—I'm unmotivated" or "I have no willpower"?

☐ Not at all likely   ☐ Slightly likely   ☐ Moderately likely   ☐ Very likely

PSYCHOLOGICAL ISSUES TOTAL _____

22. How likely are you to criticize yourself or skip meals after you've overeaten?

☐ Not at all likely   ☐ Slightly likely   ☐ Moderately likely   ☐ Very likely

23. How likely are you to say to yourself, "I've already blown it for the day so I might as well eat what I want today and start my diet again tomorrow"?

☐ Not at all likely   ☐ Slightly likely   ☐ Moderately likely   ☐ Very likely

24. How likely are you to have difficulty getting back on track the day after you've gone off track?

☐ Not at all likely   ☐ Slightly likely   ☐ Moderately likely   ☐ Very likely

GETTING OFF TRACK TOTAL _____

Building Your Escape Plan

Your journey begins with the ten foundation strategies in the next chapter. You will adopt them in order and then use these strategies as part of every escape plan. As you become more familiar with them, you'll find that you can use these skills in a variety of situations, such as getting yourself to consistently follow an exercise program—which is essential for good health, even if you didn't want to lose weight!

Losing unwanted pounds may be just the first of many changes you make in your life. *The Diet Trap Solution* teaches you to tap into the power of your mind to make change happen.

Let's get started!

Chapter 2

Foundation Strategies to Escape Your Traps

D o you want this to be the *last* time you try to lose weight? We know you're probably eager to dive headfirst into dieting so you can lose weight fast. Who wouldn't be? But we want you to think about these questions: How well has rushing into changing your eating worked for you in the long run? What does history tell you? Did you quickly lose weight—but then gain it back? Our guess is you have fallen into the same traps over and over or you wouldn't be reading this now.

Instead of focusing on how much you want to lose weight at this moment, we would like you to consider taking a longer and broader view. If you're like most people, you've been searching for the perfect diet, one that would allow you to make short-term changes so you could lose weight quickly and easily. You may not have realized that:

❶ You need an eating plan that is not only healthy, reasonable, flexible, and maintainable but also that you'll be able to follow while you're losing weight *and for as long as you want to maintain your weight loss.*

❷ You need skills to get yourself to stick to this diet while you're losing weight *and for as long as you want to maintain your weight loss,* no matter what else is going on in your life or what traps are lurking around the corner.

❸ You need to learn these strategies *before* you start following an eating plan. Day after day, you'll increase your self-discipline as you practice these strategies. And day after day, you'll increase your confidence that you can get yourself to do what you need to do, even if you don't feel like doing it. We want you to increase your self-discipline and self-confidence on easier tasks, before you tackle the much more difficult task of making lasting changes in when and what you eat.

These ten foundation strategies, first described in *The Beck Diet Solution,* vastly increase the probability that you will lose weight and keep it off. And here is the secret of success: though you'll probably be tempted, don't try to change *what* you eat right away. Instead, wait to change what you eat until you can consistently and successfully use the first eight skills. Master each skill (not just the ones you feel like learning) one by one, in the order they are presented, and you will learn *how to diet,* not just what to eat.

These ten strategies are used throughout the book because they are essential for avoiding or escaping from traps. Truthfully, if you do nothing more than use these ten universal tools consistently, you *will* lose some weight. But we also know from experience that each trap requires additional skills, specific changes in mind-set, and relevant problem solving. Taking the quiz starting on page 19 is the first step in discovering, then conquering, your own personal traps.

You don't need much preparation to start using these foundation strategies. Just some three-by-five index cards or blank business cards, copies of the foundation strategies checklist (on page 25, or downloadable at www.beckdietsolution.com), copies of the escape plan (on page 233, or downloadable at www.beckdietsolution.com), and a notebook. That's it!

Before you start, though, check out what's going through your mind. Are you already having sabotaging thoughts? You might be thinking, "This sounds like a lot of work. I have to lose weight more quickly! I can get by with just reading about the skills. I don't have to practice them."

If you're having these thoughts, we want to pose this question: What would you tell your best friend if she had struggled to lose weight and keep it off and was now asking you, "What should I do? I really want to succeed!"? Would you suggest that she not make any changes? That she continue to do what she has done in the past—even though time and again it hasn't worked in the long run?

It's time to try something different—something that will work. But if you're still not convinced, you can try an experiment. Just read the book without making any changes or use only the strategies you feel like using. Give this experiment a few weeks or months. If it works, fine! If, however, at any point you start gaining weight, we hope you'll see the necessity of instituting all these dieting skills if you really want to achieve your goal of lasting weight loss.

The ten core skills you'll use to escape your traps are contained in the foundation strategies checklist. Fill out this chart every evening. For the first few days, you will focus only on Foundation Strategy #1, and you'll have only one box to check off. Make sure you've practiced this skill for a few days or a week and have *mastered* it before adding Foundation Strategy #2. Continue like this, systematically making your way through the list and mastering the foundation strategies in the order they are presented.

Foundation Strategies Checklist

Week of: _____

	Su	M	Tu	W	Th	F	Sa
1. Read my advantages list	☐	☐	☐	☐	☐	☐	☐
2. Sat down, ate slowly, and enjoyed every bite	☐	☐	☐	☐	☐	☐	☐
3. Gave myself credit throughout the day	☐	☐	☐	☐	☐	☐	☐
4. Read my reminder cards	☐	☐	☐	☐	☐	☐	☐
5. Weighed myself	☐	☐	☐	☐	☐	☐	☐
6. Built up my resistance muscle	☐	☐	☐	☐	☐	☐	☐
7. Managed hunger and cravings	☐	☐	☐	☐	☐	☐	☐
8. Ate according to my planned schedule	☐	☐	☐	☐	☐	☐	☐
9. Followed my eating plan	☐	☐	☐	☐	☐	☐	☐
10. Created or reviewed my "worth-it memories"	☐	☐	☐	☐	☐	☐	☐

Why do you need to fill out the nightly checklist? We have found that sabotaging thoughts can really get in the way of practicing your skills. You might think, "This skill isn't really that important. I don't have to do it." Or, "I don't feel like doing it now. I'll do it later." The checklist keeps you accountable and helps you squarely face what you have and haven't done. Do you *really* want to lose weight and keep it off this time? Then it's time to make sure you're *really* practicing your skills.

Okay, ready for the first foundation strategy?

Foundation Strategy #1: Create an advantages list to motivate yourself every day. You want to lose weight for a reason—probably many incredibly important reasons. These reasons have likely occupied space in your brain for a long time. But chances are you're not able to consistently access them when you need them most: when you're tempted to eat something you shouldn't.

Think back to the last time you ate something you really regretted. Were you thinking, "I want to eat this, but I'd much rather lose weight, have more self-confidence, feel more attractive, fit into smaller-size clothes, move around more easily," and so on? Probably not, or you would have been able to resist. *This* time, though, you are going to practice reading the reasons you want to lose weight, over and over, so they are fresh in your mind when you encounter a trap. *This* time, you're going to remember why it's worth it to you to stay in control.

Make a list of all the advantages of weight loss. Maybe you'll have ten or fifteen that are highly compelling. (On the next page you'll see a sample advantages list that Jessica, the dieter you met in chapter 1, wrote.) If you would like, write each advantage on a separate card. Read the advantages every morning. Pull out the list (or the cards) as needed to boost your motivation throughout the day.

Important: *do not* just rely on trying to remember what's on the list. You undoubtedly won't be focusing on these important reasons when you get a strong craving. We've found that repeatedly reading the reasons why you want to lose weight allows you to really reflect on each one and plants them securely in your brain. Just thinking about them is not enough. So make sure you *read* them!

Jessica's Advantages List

1. I'll be more confident speaking to my boss and department heads.

2. I'll be able to wear my old clothes again, especially shorts and skirts.

3. I'll start wearing colors again, not just black, and I'll enjoy shopping for clothes like I used to.

4. I'll be able to walk up steps without getting winded.

5. I'll enjoy dancing at parties and weddings.

6. I'll do more activities, like kayaking and hiking, with Josh.

7. I'll avoid developing diabetes.

8. I'll feel proud of myself.

9. I won't be at the mercy of cravings and negative emotions.

10. I'll feel good about looking in the mirror and having photographs taken.

Here are some ideas to keep the advantages fresh: Shuffle the deck from time to time. Rearrange the deck so the ones that feel most significant to you that day are on top. Visualize, in detail, achieving each advantage and how good you'll feel. Enter the list on your personal electronic device. Set pop-ups on your computer or phone throughout the day with a different reason each time.

Creating your advantages list and repeatedly reviewing it

- **Helps you focus on the payoffs** for all the time and effort you're putting into dieting, instead of what you're "giving up."

- **Cements the reasons more firmly in your mind** for the times when you get blindsided by a trap. Every time you read the cards, you are strengthening your neural pathways and helping rewire your brain's automatic thinking.

Foundation Strategy #2: Sit down, eat slowly, and enjoy every bite. Ultimately, you will probably be taking fewer bites than you are right now, so we want you to learn how to get maximum satisfaction from each one. This skill may be a little harder than you think, if you're used to eating quickly without being aware of each bite. You may even be like a number of dieters who sometimes try not to notice what they're eating because if they did they would feel guilty.

You simply can't pay enough attention to your food if you're not sitting down, and you rob yourself of full enjoyment. Unfortunately, when you eat standing up, you usually eat without full awareness, so you don't derive as much satisfaction. Feeling unsatisfied can then drive you to eat more. In fact, you can easily consume hundreds of extra calories a day (if not more) when you eat standing up. You may "graze" while standing in front of the refrigerator or food cabinets. Maybe you eat as you're taking food to and from the table or putting away leftovers. Perhaps you take free samples of food at markets or fairs. Somehow you fool yourself into thinking that this kind of eating "doesn't count." But of course it does! Every calorie adds up.

It's also difficult to fully pay attention to what you're eating when you're distracted, whether you're watching television or surfing the web or reading a magazine. On the other hand, engaging in conversation with your dining companions can also be distracting. You don't need to eliminate these distractions, but you do need to train yourself to fully focus on your food by eating alone for a few meals, with no distractions.

Once you've mastered that step, reintroduce the distractions. A visual cue (such as a different place mat) or an auditory cue (such as a periodic tone on a smartphone timer app) can remind you to ask yourself, "Have I been paying attention to my food for the last few bites?" If not, put your utensils down, have a sip of water, and start again. Also consider taking smaller bites. You can eat a slice of apple pie in five bites, but if you eat it in fifteen bites, you get ten additional bites to enjoy.

Eating sitting down, slowly and mindfully,

- **Makes you aware of how much you're actually eating.** No longer will you find yourself mindlessly eating one chip after another.

- **Increases your enjoyment of food.** You'll be able to more fully experience the flavors and textures of what you're eating so you get a bigger bang for your buck.

- **Leads to greater psychological satisfaction.** When you see all the food you're going to eat spread out on the table in front of you, you'll feel more gratified than if you miss this visual display by eating one food after another standing up.

- **Provides greater physical satisfaction.** When you eat slowly, you give your brain a chance to register satiety before you overeat. Additionally, being aware of every bite you take helps you feel full and satisfied. We simply don't feel as satisfied, physically or psychologically, by bites we barely remember eating.

Foundation Strategy #3: Give yourself credit each time you practice a skill or make a positive food choice. To be successful, you need to increase your sense of "self-efficacy," a strong belief in your ability to do what you need to do. Take special notice and praise yourself ("That's good! I deserve credit for that!") every time you use a foundation strategy, such as reading your advantages list (and extra credit if you didn't feel like doing it but did it anyway) or resisting an extra helping of macaroni and cheese. Set up a reminder system to monitor yourself throughout the day, such as a note on your schedule, a pop-up on your computer screen, or an alarm on your phone.

This skill is critical. Some dieters believe they don't deserve credit until they actually lose weight. But then they miss out on all the surprising benefits of using this strategy. Giving yourself credit

- **Helps motivate you.** You *deserve* pats on the back every time you practice a skill and make a healthy eating decision.

- **Helps you keep mistakes in perspective.** If you're like most of the dieters we've worked with, you tend to focus on the one or two mistakes you make in a day or a week and forget about all the things you have done well. Giving yourself credit helps reverse this trend and lets you view your experience more realistically—unlike the distorted view you get when you pay attention only to the negatives.

- **Helps you get back on track.** If you've been hearing, "That's good!" all day, you'll realize, "Yes, I ate an extra roll at dinner, but I also did twenty other things right today. No big deal. It was just one mistake." It will be easier to get back in control immediately, instead of making a lot more mistakes.

- **Helps get you through the difficult times.** You need self-confidence when the going gets tough so you won't give up. Recognizing all the positive changes you're making in your thinking and your behavior gives you evidence, over and over again, that you have what it takes to lose weight. The more evidence you accumulate, the more certain you will become that you can keep on going.

- **Helps you realize that losing weight isn't a fluke.** In the past, when you started to gain weight back, you may have said, "I don't know how I lost weight in the first place," which most likely led to a nosedive in your confidence and decreased your motivation to begin again. On the other hand, if you've consistently recognized and credited yourself for practicing your skills and making good eating choices, you'll be able to say, "I know exactly how I lost weight and what I need to do to start losing again."

> **Warning: Don't skip this strategy! It's easy to forget to practice this skill throughout the day. What keeps successful dieters and maintainers going is giving themselves credit.**

Foundation Strategy #4: Create "reminder cards" to respond to your sabotaging thoughts. Once you start looking, you will probably find that you have lots of sabotaging thinking that leads you to give in to temptation. Composing and then regularly reading compelling responses prepares you for traps you may encounter throughout the day.

Some of your sabotaging thoughts will begin, "It's okay to eat this [food] I hadn't planned because . . ." and end in any number of unproductive ways:

"I'm happy/sad/tired/celebrating."

"It's free."

"No one is watching."

"I'm at a party."

"I have to get my money's worth."

"It has healthy ingredients in it."

"I hardly ever get to have it."

"I'll exercise later."

"I've been so good all day."

"I can't waste food."

Now imagine if you'd been reading the following reminder card regularly:

I need to face reality. If my goal is to lose weight, it's <u>not</u> okay to eat unplanned food. I can always plan to eat it tomorrow, but history has taught me that making spontaneous decisions to go off my plan just doesn't work. When I get on the scale tomorrow, I'm going to be very glad I didn't eat it.

This card, plus many others that you'll make, will help keep you on track in tempting situations. This is how to create them:

❶ Every morning, look ahead to the day. Ask yourself, "What challenging eating situations (traps) will I encounter? What might go through my mind that could lead me astray? What do I want to be able to tell myself in those situations?"

❷ Whenever you regret something you've eaten, ask yourself, "What did I tell myself that led me to eat something I wasn't supposed to eat? How do I wish I had answered that thought?"

Write your responses on cards or use a note-taking program or app on your smartphone. If you have difficulty composing a compelling response, don't worry. We will provide lots of ideas.

Read your reminder cards every morning, and pull them out just before you enter a tempting situation. If you encounter a surprise temptation,

excuse yourself, go to a private spot, and review your cards again. Learning to create reminder cards and developing the self-discipline to read
them daily are essential prerequisites for creating effective escape plans.

You can even use this technique if you have sabotaging thoughts that
interfere with practicing the skills you're learning about in this book—for
example, "It's okay if I don't practice my foundation strategies because . . .
I'm too busy. I don't really need them. I don't feel like doing them."

Creating reminder cards

- **Helps you anticipate sabotaging thoughts** you're likely to have and
  prepare for them in advance.

- **Allows you to practice your new ideas.** Just as simply thinking
  about the advantages of losing weight isn't sufficient, it's also not
  enough to mentally rehearse helpful ways of thinking. You need
  to focus and reflect on compelling responses to your sabotaging
  thoughts so you can stop fooling yourself, especially when you think
  you can avoid practicing your skills or go off your eating plan and
  still lose weight.

- **Gives you a replacement habit for vulnerable times.** Sometimes
  it's helpful to give your brain something to do while a craving
  passes. Physically holding on to the cards gives your body a sensory
  reminder of your long-term goals.

Foundation Strategy #5: Weigh yourself daily. Does this rec-
ommendation surprise you? Perhaps you've heard that you should only
weigh yourself once a week. We'd like to explain why this is a crucial
foundation strategy.

When dieters first come to see us, we find that many avoid weighing themselves, at least on some days, especially when they're worried
they've gained weight and don't want to face the consequences of their
eating. It's much easier to maintain control in the face of temptation when
you know you will absolutely get on the scale the next morning.

Many people find it problematic to weigh themselves only once a week
because *the number on the scale does not always correspond to what you ate
the day before.* Has this happened to you? You were "perfect" on your
diet one day, but you find your weight has gone up by two pounds the
next morning. Maybe you had hormonal changes, retained water, got less

sleep, or experienced some unidentified physiological change. The truth is, the scale should *not* go down every day—or even every week. Weight loss just doesn't work that way. But if your weigh-in day was the one day all week when your weight was temporarily up, you might feel discouraged and put yourself at risk for giving up. Weighing yourself daily allows you to get accustomed to the scale's normal fluctuations.

Weigh yourself each morning before breakfast. Get on the scale just once and that's it! You can decide whether to record your weight in your notebook (or using an app) on a daily or weekly basis. Just make sure to be consistent, whatever you choose.

If you're tempted not to weigh yourself at all, you can make a reminder card with some reasons why this skill is essential.

Weighing yourself daily

- **Helps you disregard unexplained weight gain on any given day.** It can be difficult to avoid feeling discouraged when your weight is up, especially if you're accustomed to weighing yourself once a week. You'll quickly learn to take the long view when you weigh yourself daily because you will have seven times as many opportunities to confirm that fluctuations are normal and that the scale does go down over time.

- **Makes you more accountable every day.** You'll find it much easier to stick to your eating plan when you know that deviating from it could show up on the scale tomorrow.

- **Helps desensitize you to the number on the scale.** The more often you weigh yourself, the more opportunities you have to recognize that your weight is just a number—and not a reflection of who you are.

Foundation Strategy #6: Build up your "resistance muscle." Here's a common sabotaging thought that often precedes a dieting mistake: *It's okay if I make an exception this one time. It won't matter.* The implication is that there won't be any consequences for eating something you weren't supposed to eat.

But there is a consequence—a major one. Every time you make an exception, you make it more likely that the *next time* you'll also make an exception—and the time after that and the time after that. Each exception strengthens what we call your psychological "giving-in muscle" and undermines your confidence in your ability to stick to a plan. To succeed at weight loss and maintenance, you need a very weak giving-in muscle.

On the other hand, every time you're tempted to go off plan but you don't, you strengthen your "resistance muscle," and you also increase your confidence that you *can* resist. You start to create an image of yourself as a person who can stand strong in the face of temptation, which makes it easier to resist the next time and the time after that and the time after that.

So every time you respond to the temptation to make an exception, you either strengthen your giving-in muscle and weaken your resistance muscle *or* you strengthen your resistance muscle and weaken your giving-in muscle. That's why *every time matters,* whether your decision is to skip a strategy or to eat something you're not supposed to.

No matter what goal you have for yourself in life, the more confident you are that you can get yourself to do what you need to do, the easier it will be to work toward that goal and the more likely you are to achieve it.

Our dieters get to the point where they're *glad* that they passed up extra food and stayed in control. Researchers from the University of Chicago reported a similar finding.[4] People felt a boost in mood when they successfully resisted a temptation, *even at the very moment* they were "depriving" themselves. When you stay in control, you feel proud of yourself

> Every decision matters. If I choose to make an exception, I'll strengthen my giving-in muscle and weaken my resistance muscle, and it will get harder and harder to avoid exceptions in the future. If I decide to stay in control, I'll strengthen my resistance muscle and weaken my giving-in muscle, and it will get easier and easier to make good choices in the future. Every time matters.

and relieved that you're no longer struggling with the to-eat-or-not-to-eat decision.

Think about how many exceptions you've made in the past and how they have affected your weight. Create a reminder card, such as the one on the previous page, to read daily so you can practice a compelling response to self-talk that tells you an exception doesn't matter. You may fool yourself by thinking, "It's only pretzel crumbs. Can't be more than twenty calories." But it's not just the calories that should be your primary concern—*it's the habit*.

Strengthening your resistance muscle

- **Helps you develop the self-control you need to lose weight.** Success builds on success. Having a well-developed resistance muscle will make dieting much easier.

- **Prepares you for difficult times ahead.** Using your foundation strategies generally makes dieting—and later, maintenance—go relatively smoothly. But there will always be traps. A strong resistance muscle will keep you out of them!

Foundation Strategy #7: Manage hunger and cravings. If you have been trying to be careful with your eating as you were mastering the first six skills, you have probably experienced hunger and cravings. If you gave in and ate more than you should have, don't beat yourself up! You haven't yet learned all the skills you need.

Ultimately, you'll learn that you don't have to do *anything* about hunger or cravings. Once you start eating according to a schedule (the next foundation strategy), you'll find what all successful dieters and maintainers know: that hunger and cravings reach a peak and then subside. They don't just get worse and worse and worse until you can't tolerate them any longer.

We ask our dieters (except those who can't fast for several hours for a medical reason) to do the hunger and cravings experiment. Afterward, they often tell us that this experiment has turned out to be one of the most liberating experiences of their lives because it has helped them finally believe, both at an intellectual and an emotional level, that they *never again* have to worry about hunger or cravings.

The Hunger and Cravings Experiment

This experiment has three steps:

1. Create a "discomfort scale" in your notebook. Write down at least one experience for each level of discomfort, such as in the following example:

Severe Physical Discomfort	Moderate Physical Discomfort	Mild Physical Discomfort
After surgery	Migraine headache	Run-of-the-mill stomachache

2. Choose one day and eat a good, satiating breakfast—and then don't eat again until dinner. (Sip water for thirst but don't try to fill up by drinking.)

3. Set a timer to go off every hour on the hour. When it does, look at your discomfort scale and ask yourself, "How physically uncomfortable do I feel right now (because of hunger or cravings)?" and, "What was the range of discomfort I felt in the previous hour?" Write down the time and your answers to these two questions in your notebook.

If you're like other dieters, you'll discover that hunger and cravings are almost never more than mildly uncomfortable, and they disappear, usually after several minutes, especially if you focus on something else. Even when they reappear, they very rarely get to the point of moderate discomfort. By doing this experiment, you will prove to yourself that you can absolutely tolerate the intermittent, mild discomfort of hunger and cravings because you have tolerated far greater discomfort in your life.

Ideally, from now on, whenever you want to eat something you know you shouldn't, you'll just accept the mild, short-lived discomfort of not eating it, and you'll automatically turn your attention to something else. But you may need an interim step: deliberate distraction. On a card (or on your phone, if you carry it all the time), create a list of activities that will compellingly engage your mind. You may need one list with activities you can do at home and another for activities you can do at work.

Here is Jessica's list.

Distraction List

Take a walk
Call Ezra, Maya, or Tom
Write e-mails
Surf the web
Watch funny YouTube videos
Play game on phone
Clean out desk drawer or closet shelf
Do a crossword puzzle
Give myself a manicure or facial

Continue to add to the list as you think of other activities. Then, when you encounter a trap, engage in one activity after another until the urge to eat subsides.

Managing your hunger and cravings

- **Helps keep you on track.** When temptation hits, you'll be able to tell yourself, "Big deal. It's just an urge to eat. It will go away."

- **Increases your confidence.** When you get really good at this skill, you won't have to fear potential traps! You'll know that you can definitely accept the mild discomfort of not eating.

Foundation Strategy #8: Eat according to a schedule. Do you know when most dieters run into trouble? When they make spontaneous decisions about whether to eat something. These spontaneous decisions are rarely to eat *less* than they had planned; the decisions are almost always to eat more.

Have you ever promised yourself that you're not going to eat until a certain time? Then you encounter some mouth-watering food (at a store, a get-together, a meeting, or a vending machine). And you impulsively eat it, because you haven't mastered eating according to a schedule.

Here's what to do: First, focus on planning *when* you're going to eat, not *what* you're going to eat. (That's the next foundation strategy.) There's no magic schedule. Experiment to find what works best for you. Maybe you'll do well with breakfast, snack, lunch, snack, dinner, snack. Some dieters prefer just three meals a day, with no snacks. Others like having three meals plus two snacks after dinner. Remember, the best schedule is the one you can successfully maintain. You can give yourself a range (of up to about two hours) for each meal and snack. Here is the schedule that suited Jessica best:

> **Breakfast** between 7:30 and 8:30
>
> **Lunch** between 12:00 and 2:00
>
> **Afternoon snack** between 3:00 and 4:30
>
> **Dinner** between 5:30 and 7:30
>
> **Dessert** between 8:00 and 9:30

Eating according to a schedule

- **Reduces the struggle** over eating. No more asking, "Should I eat this? Shouldn't I?" If it's not time to eat, you don't eat.

- **Eliminates spontaneous eating.** Making impulsive decisions about when to eat has probably been a downfall in the past. Once you master eating according to a schedule, you'll find that it's much easier to stay on plan.

Foundation Strategy #9: Adopt (and adapt) an eating plan you can follow *for life*. You absolutely need a reasonable, flexible, nutritious diet if you want to escape your traps, lose weight, and maintain weight loss. You won't have long-term success with an unhealthy or overly restrictive diet.

Why, you ask? If eating fewer calories than you burn is the basis of any weight-loss plan, why can't you just drastically reduce your calories and lose weight quickly?

Answer: *There is no such thing as cutting calories in the short term and then increasing calories without gaining weight.* In fact, we don't want dieters to make changes they can't keep up for life, unless they are under the care of a medical provider. The changes you make to lose weight are exactly the same changes you need to maintain weight loss. Dieting and maintenance are identical. No more "three [excruciating] weeks to a new body!" diet plans. That's a recipe for eventual failure. You need to think long term.

We don't recommend specific diets because people vary in the foods they consider healthy, appealing, and sustainable. Current research shows that some diets lead to greater weight loss than other diets—but it's usually a matter of eight pounds versus six pounds—a pretty minimal difference.[5] So the best diet is one that's healthy and that you can stick to—and that has a truly sustainable calorie level, given your lifestyle and appetite.

Your eating plan has to provide proper nutrition. Don't fool yourself into thinking you can eat whatever you want as long as you don't go over a certain calorie count for the day. Some foods (especially protein, fats, and fiber) minimize hunger. Other foods (especially processed carbs and sugar) make you feel hungry much sooner and can lead to cravings. And if you're not eating a balanced diet, you'll run into health problems sooner or later.

Most of our dieters tend to increase the amount of lean protein, whole grains, fruits, and vegetables they eat and make sure to eat a moderate amount of healthy fat. That's what keeps them full and satisfied. They also tend to reduce their intake of processed food and carbs and caloric beverages. But they don't entirely eliminate any food.

And here's an important caveat: you may need to tweak the eating plan you choose if it doesn't include your favorite foods. If you love bread, we know you're going to end up eating bread again at some point in your life—and we want you to! There's no reason to eliminate it, now or ever. You just need to learn the skills, presented in this chapter and throughout the book, to limit your consumption of certain foods.

Remember, we don't want you to make any changes in your eating that you can't keep up. It is completely unrealistic to think that you can eliminate your favorite foods long term. Many of our dieters decide to have one reasonable portion of junk food every day. They usually plan to eat it in the evening, so they can look forward to it all day long. Avoiding junk food at other times is much easier because they think, "Even though I'd like to eat that cookie now, I'm going to resist because I'd much rather have the candy bar that's on my plan for after dinner." And planning a treat every night also keeps them from eating more than one portion because they know they can have it (or another junk food item) the next day and the next day and the next, for the rest of their lives.

Make sure your eating plan is flexible. You can't always control the food that's available, especially if you're not eating at home. So you need an eating plan that will allow you to eat reasonable portions of whatever is served.

In the evening, write down what you intend to eat the next day (or write it down each morning for the current day). Record what, how much, and when you'll eat. Then, as you go through your day, check off what you've eaten and write in capital letters anything you ate that you weren't supposed to so you can honestly face your mistakes and figure out what you need to do differently next time.

You won't have to write out a food plan forever. Once you learn how to stay out of traps, you'll be able to make a mental plan. You'll figure out which foods work best for you and which portion sizes allow you to continue losing weight or maintain your weight loss.

Adapting a healthy, well-balanced plan that's right for you, deciding in advance what to eat, and monitoring your eating as you go along

- **Keeps you nourished.** A nutritious diet not only supplies the nutrients you need but also minimizes hunger and cravings.

- **Helps you resist urges to eat food you'll later regret.** Even if you can't eat a food that's calling your name at the moment, you can always plan to have it the next day.

- **Increases your accountability.** When you know you will have to write down whatever you spontaneously eat, you're far less likely to eat off plan.

Foundation Strategy #10: Capture "worth-it memories" to remind you why it's worth it to you to stick to your plan. Unsuccessful dieters tend to give up when the going gets tough. A key sabotaging thought is "It isn't worth all this effort." That's why it's essential to build a storehouse of memories that remind you why it *is* worth it: memories of the times you felt really happy that you stayed in control. Such experiences might include:

- When someone compliments you on your new appearance

- When you fit into smaller-size clothing

- When your weight goes down

- When you move more gracefully and with greater ease

- When you feel more confident around other people

- When you fit more comfortably in your seat at the movies, in a plane, or in an amusement park ride

- When you have a great time at an event because you followed your eating plan and felt in control

- When you return home from vacation and feel good about getting on the scale

Keep a "worth-it memories" section in your notebook, create an entirely new memory journal to capture these accomplishments, or write these experiences on index cards or on an electronic device. Perhaps best of all would be a diary app that provides you with the opportunity to write about these situations and to include a photo or video that captures the experience. Read through your memories at least once a week when dieting is easier and once a day when dieting gets harder.

Here is an entry that Jessica composed:

May 5

I feel great! I went to Abigail's party and I stayed in control. I had one piece of cake, just as I had planned, and then I stopped. I really enjoyed the cake because I ate it slowly and enjoyed every bite—and completely without guilt. I was tempted to eat a second piece but I reminded myself that it wasn't worth it and that I wouldn't enjoy it anyway because I'd feel guilty about it. I left the party feeling proud; it's a great feeling. It was totally worth it.

Capturing "worth-it memories":

- **Increases your pleasure and pride.** As you focus on these positive situations, you prolong the experience and the positive emotions that come from the awareness that you've stayed in control of your eating.

- **Increases your motivation when the going gets tough.** Reviewing these personally meaningful and important memories allows you to visualize and relive these positive moments at a deep level. Remembering how good those moments felt creates a warm feeling of accomplishment that will give you energy to keep going, especially when staying in control is difficult, so you can achieve your goal of lasting weight loss.

Putting It All Together: How to Create Escape Plans

At the end of each trap chapter, you'll devise a personalized escape plan for specific situations you expect to encounter. You will find a blank escape plan template in the appendix, or at www.beckdietsolution.com, so you can make copies. For each trap, identify each situation that is likely to arise and create an escape plan for each one. Here are the steps to create your escape plan:

❶ **Specify the trap at the top.**

❷ **Describe a specific situation in which this trap might arise.**
For example:

- *Super Bowl party at Daniel and Hillary's—they'll expect me to eat and drink a lot.*

- *All-you-can-eat buffet when we go out with the kids. I'll be tempted to eat too much.*

- *Feeling anxious about the results of my blood test. I'll want to soothe myself with food.*

- *Not enough time to eat lunch on Friday, so I'll have the urge to snack throughout the afternoon.*

❸ **Record your sabotaging thoughts.** What could go through your mind when you're in this situation? Here are two examples of Jessica's thoughts:

- *It's Molly's wedding. I should enjoy myself and eat and drink whatever I want.*

- *I should be able to eat whatever Ethan is eating.*

Review the relevant traps in the chapter to see if there are additional thoughts you are likely to have that you should add to the chart.

❹ **Write a compelling response to each sabotaging thought.** For ideas, look through the reminder cards you've already created and review relevant material in the current chapter and other chapters. You can also imagine what you would say to a friend who was in the same situation.

Jessica answered her sabotaging thoughts this way:

- *If I stay on plan, I'll leave the wedding feeling great. I'll feel so proud of myself.*

- *If I want to lose weight, I have to get really good at sticking to my plan. What Ethan is eating is irrelevant. He doesn't have a goal to lose weight like I do. I can always plan to eat what he's having tomorrow, though probably in smaller portions.*

If you get stuck and can't create a compelling response, ask a friend or fellow dieters on an online forum for help.

❺ **Develop a list of strategies.** In the third column, write down techniques you can use. Refer to any relevant chapter, especially this chapter. As you're filling in this column, be on the lookout for additional sabotaging thoughts:

- *I know I should get up from the table and go read my advantages list but I don't feel like it.*

Add them—and strong responses to them—to the first and second columns in your chart.

❻ **Review your escape plan often.** You are so much more likely to escape this trap if you read—and perhaps add to—your escape plan repeatedly before the situation arises.

❼ **Revise your escape plan.** After the situation is over, evaluate how well the escape plan worked. Were your reminders strong enough? Did you have additional sabotaging thoughts? Do you need extra strategies? Modify the escape plan so it will be more helpful the next time you need it.

At this point, you will have a fully completed escape plan. You can transfer the reminders to reminder cards and strategies to an actual or virtual strategies list, or you can just keep reviewing your escape plan as is. In fact, even if you find that the portability of cards works better for you, continue to periodically review your escape plans. You may find that some sabotaging thoughts pop up in different traps, and many of the strategies you've devised will also apply to other traps.

As you create, revise, and review your escape plans, you'll internalize a new mind-set, and you'll arm yourself with effective strategies. Writing down your escape plans and having everything spelled out vastly increases the probability that you'll remember and commit to the changes you need to make so you can attain your goal of losing weight and keeping it off.

Are You Ready?

Okay! Now that you're armed with the ten foundation strategies and the instructions for creating your escape plans, turn to the chapters that correspond to your highest scores on the "What Are Your Biggest Traps?" quiz starting on page 19. Read through each of the personal stories, paying close attention to the situations and sabotaging thoughts that resonate with you. At the end of each chapter, you'll put the lessons of these stories to work in your own life by creating an escape plan for each difficult situation you expect to encounter. Continue to read through the book to learn additional strategies and keep refining your escape plans. You'll understand in a very personal way how universal your struggle is and how effective escape plans can be in overcoming your traps.

The strategies to get out of the traps—and stay out—are powerful. Using them consistently will allow you to finally achieve your goal of lasting weight loss. And the strategies can be adapted to help you achieve other goals that are important and meaningful to you.

It's time to free yourself from your traps—for good!

PART TWO

Internal Traps:
How I Trap Myself

Chapter 3

Stress Traps

U nless you are properly prepared to escape them, stress traps aren't just bumps on the weight-loss road; they're sinkholes that can swallow you whole. Stress is often the destroyer of good intentions. How many times have you heard yourself say, "I'm too busy to go to the store. I'll just grab some fast food for dinner" or "I'm too stressed out right now to think about healthy eating. I'll start working on it next week"?

We find it baffling that *all* diet programs don't help dieters prepare for and counteract stress. "Just follow the program," they say. But to be successful, you need to know what to do when you inevitably encounter demanding and hectic days, weeks, or even months. How can you get through these difficult periods without letting stress traps derail your healthy eating efforts? You need to learn how to problem-solve, prioritize your activities, respond to your sabotaging thinking, and take care of yourself, so you'll have the time and energy it takes to stay on track.

Chances are you have dozens of personal stories of stress ("Everything was fine until X happened") that impeded your efforts to lose weight. Consider the experiences of the dieters in this chapter and see if they ring a bell. These dieters were able to decrease their stress—and you can, too, once you learn how.

#1: The Too Busy Trap

Your life feels too packed and stressful to make time for healthy eating.

Miranda was a single mother of two boys, one in elementary and one in middle school. She worked full time at a clothing store while she was studying for her bachelor's degree. When she first came to see me, she didn't have to say she was stressed; it was written all over her face.

Miranda rushed in ten minutes late with a cell phone glued to her ear. "Sorry," she said as she hung up. "My son is sick, and I had to find someone to pick him up from school." As she spoke, her cell buzzed again. She told her mother she would call her back in an hour.

Several years before, Miranda had gone through a painful divorce, a major catalyst for her weight gain. "I kind of fell apart, to be honest," she told me, as she shredded a tissue. "That's when I began overeating. I'd always weighed about the same since high school, but I started gaining. Now I'm up seventy pounds, and it hasn't stopped."

She looked out the window. "Most days I feel like a chicken with its head cut off. I'm so stressed—I can't even believe I made it here."

Stress is an inevitable part of life. Most people can flourish under moderate stress. Positive stress can keep life exciting, motivating and challenging us to accomplish our goals. Athletes, actors, stock traders, and other peak performers all talk about thriving on the adrenaline rush. But for many, like Miranda, stress can become chronic and negative, especially when it stems from financial challenges, overwhelming responsibilities, lack of emotional or physical support, relationship or work difficulties, or illness.

Miranda felt her stress level rise each morning as soon as she got out of bed and had to face the day. The daily grind of traffic, work, school, and family obligations continued the pressure through the day, and she scrambled even more if one of her kids was sick. On most days, by the time she picked up the boys from their after-school program and brought them home, it was nearly seven o'clock. Everyone was so hungry that dinner was usually pizza or fast food she picked up on the way home.

Miranda was accustomed to eating many meals standing up while talking on the phone, going through mail, or doing chores. Sometimes she just grazed and didn't take time to eat a real meal at all. Once she started, Miranda often continued to eat throughout the evening, nibbling on leftovers and whatever snacks she had in the house—which were usually not very nutritious.

"I know it's bad not just for me but also for the kids," she said. The nurses at school had sent notes home a couple of months before that said what Miranda already knew: both boys were overweight. She knew she wasn't setting a good example. "Their health, and my health, are the main reasons I want to change how we eat," she said. "But I don't know how to do it, and there aren't enough hours in the day."

Miranda started learning Foundation Strategy #1 in our first session. Reading her advantages list each morning was no sweat, and she also found it easy to review her reminder cards every day and to give herself credit. But when I introduced the skill of eating everything sitting down, slowly and mindfully, she hesitated. Miranda understood the idea—in theory. She recognized that since she would ultimately be eating less food than she might desire, mastering the skill of noticing and enjoying each bite would help her maximize her satisfaction.

She expressed some reservations. "I don't think I'll have time to eat breakfast sitting down," she said. "I usually just grab a muffin and eat it while I clear up the dishes and make sure the boys have packed their backpacks." Miranda's lunchtime was booked with running errands for herself and her boys. And I had already heard about her multitasking at dinnertime. If she was to succeed, Miranda needed to find a way to make healthy eating a top priority, or it would just never happen in the context of her busy life. At least for the time being, something needed to change.

Looking at her schedule, we saw a number of things she did on a regular basis that were certainly desirable but not necessarily *essential*. To sit down for meals, Miranda clearly needed to dedicate some time in the evening and on weekends to chores she usually did in the morning and during dinner. And she also needed time for self-care to recharge her batteries. We brainstormed a few options. By setting her alarm half an hour earlier, Miranda could prepare a reasonable breakfast, eat slowly and mindfully with the boys, and still have time to make sure they were ready for school. She solved the breakfast cleanup problem by assigning this chore to her sons. From now on, they would put the food away, load the dishes in the dishwasher, and wipe off the table. Then we looked at other tasks she could eliminate, reduce, or delegate, for a short time at least. We came up with a good plan, but next we needed to identify whether sabotaging thoughts might get in the way.

Miranda realized that when the alarm went off half an hour earlier, she might think, "I don't really need to get up right now. I can just rush through breakfast like I usually do; it will be okay." After thinking it through, Miranda concluded that getting up at the last minute and grabbing whatever she could for breakfast reduced her satisfaction, reinforced negative eating habits, and provided a poor example to her kids. She made the following reminder card:

> When the alarm goes off in the morning, remember: rushing through breakfast has *never* helped me lose weight. If I stay in bed, I won't enjoy the time anyway because I'll spend it feeling guilty about not getting up. Plus I want to be a good role model. So just get up *now!*

Next I suggested that Miranda envision asking her sons to do the breakfast cleanup. Her mother guilt kicked in. She said, "I don't think it's fair to ask them to do extra work just because I need to lose weight." Sabotaging thought! As we talked about another way of looking at the situation, Miranda realized that having her sons take part in household chores would actually be positive. Her reminder card read:

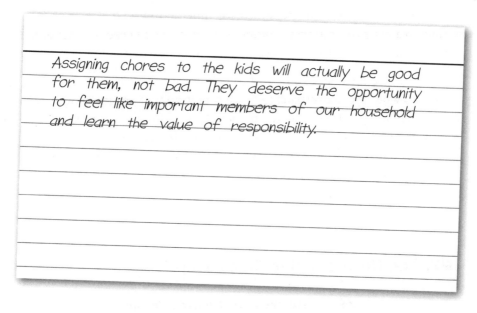

Assigning chores to the kids will actually be good for them, not bad. They deserve the opportunity to feel like important members of our household and learn the value of responsibility.

With these two changes in her family's morning schedule, Miranda was on her way to reducing her stress level for the day.

Escape the Too Busy Trap

Often the most successful escape from the too busy trap includes recognizing that you are human and have limits. Reconsidering your priorities and delegating tasks to others can be immensely freeing.

- If you want to be able to lose weight, you have to fit the rest of your life around healthy eating, not try to fit it into an already packed day.

- Consider your daily schedule. Look for tasks you are doing that you could, at least temporarily,

  cut back on *(Can you do less volunteering for a few weeks?);*

  do less well *(Do you really need to have a completely spotless house?);* or

  stop doing *(How about having the kids take the bus to school instead of driving them?).*

Your goal requires an investment of time and energy. You can't add water to a glass that's already completely full. You will need to pour some out to make room for *you* in your life. It will be worth it!

- Ask yourself, whom can I enlist to help me get things done? Sometimes when we're overwhelmed, we find it difficult to stop long enough to see who can lend a helping hand. Think of your family, your friends, your neighbors, your kids' friends' parents, your coworkers. People are often happy, or at least willing, to help, but if you don't ask, you won't receive.

#2: The Unreasonable Rules Trap

You create overly restrictive rules for yourself that lead to stress.

Miranda agreed that it was practical for her to do nonessential errands on the weekend, but she didn't know how she would fit this in. "My Saturdays and Sundays are already jam-packed. I have schoolwork to do, and housework, and marketing, and I try to go to all the games and practices for both boys."

I said, "Let me ask you this: What if you had kidney trouble and had to go to dialysis every Saturday and Sunday for at least an hour? Would you find time for that?"

"Of course!"

"That means if you *absolutely* had to fit something else into your weekends, you could do it, no question." Miranda nodded. We figured out that she could free up considerable time if she modified her usual plan of going to every soccer and basketball practice and staying for the entire time. We came up with some options:

- She could simply drop them off and pick them up.

- She could return for only the final half hour.

- She could get someone else, such as her brother, to drive them (and maybe stay and watch, too).

"I don't know," she sighed. "I'd really feel guilty."

I wondered aloud whether Miranda held herself to an unhelpful standard of doing everything she possibly could for her sons. She thought a moment, then admitted that she felt as if she had to give 110 percent to make up for the divorce and make sure her boys were okay. Even when she realized that the boys would benefit from spending more time with her brother, Adam, another unhelpful rule interfered: "I should do everything myself."

Unreasonable rules like these add stress to an already challenging situation. You, too, may have unhelpful expectations that you're not fully aware of. Miranda clearly needed to see her situation from a different perspective. "I wonder what you'd say to your best friend if she were in the same situation?" I asked.

Miranda pondered the question. "I guess I'd tell Sonya that if her goal is to lose weight and be healthier, she has to make some changes, even if it affects her kids."

"And if she protested? If she said, 'I *should* go to all my kids' events. I *should* do everything myself,' what would you tell her?"

Miranda let out a deep sigh. "I'd tell her that her health is more important. That it would be nice to be able to go to every single one of the boys' events, but she shouldn't—at least for now. Because getting healthy will be better for her kids than going to every game."

Miranda realized that she needed to take her own advice. She made this reminder card:

> If I want to be healthy and want the kids to be healthy, I have to make healthy eating a top priority. The boys might be disappointed if I don't go to all their practices and games, but they'll get over it. And it would be good to get Adam more involved in their lives.

Next we discussed a new standard. Miranda saw the wisdom in changing her 110 percent rule to a more moderate one: "I should be a good mom and also take care of myself." But it was still hard for her to imagine actually doing less for the boys. I reminded her how parents on an airplane are directed to first put on their own oxygen masks, so they can be in shape to then help their children. "If you pass out," I reminded her, "you're no good to the person next to you!"

Miranda thought about how this concept applied to her life. She decided that her new rule should actually be phrased, "I should be a good mom but I *have* to take care of myself to *be* a good mom." This new guideline helped her find breathing space in her life. For example, instead of waiting until the last minute and scrambling to pull something together for dinner, she would use the time while Adam was with the boys to plan meals for the week and shop for healthy ingredients. She would reserve a little time on Sundays to chop vegetables for the week and make at least part of her sons' lunches (which would help them eat healthier). She enlisted the boys' help, and the three of them started a new tradition of spending time together in the kitchen.

With these key activities pushed to the top of the list, Miranda's life started to settle down a bit. We continued to look for stress-relieving tweaks to her schedule—especially self-care. With her new rule in mind, Miranda carved out a little time to have coffee with friends, read, and watch TV. When she felt stressed or rushed, she practiced a mindfulness technique, listening to a five-minute recording on her smartphone that helped her focus on her breathing. This technique made her feel more relaxed and calm.

These changes did the trick. At our last visit, Miranda had lost twenty-six pounds and was still on the way down. She was so proud of herself for getting her eating—and her sons' eating—under control. "But losing weight and getting healthier is only half the story," she related. "My stress is way down. I feel like I can breathe again for the first time in years."

Escape the Unreasonable Rules Trap

Without even realizing it, you may impose expectations on yourself that make your stress exponentially worse. Life is hard enough without putting arbitrary measures of performance on top of already stressful situations.

- Think about whether you have unreasonable rules for yourself. Usually these sabotaging thoughts incorporate *should* or *have to* or *need to* and an absolute word, such as *always* or *every* or *never:* "I have to always make my family happy. I should never do less than my absolute best at work."

- Ask yourself, "What would I say to [a specific friend or family member] if she were in my situation and had the same rule for herself?" You'd likely have a more reasonable perspective. Deep down you probably know what would be best for her—and for yourself. Then take your own advice.

#3: The De-Stress with Food Trap

You eat to relax after a stressful day.

Greg was a private security officer who struggled under a heavy burden of stress. His main motivation for weight loss was more than thirty pounds of excess bulk that he carried around his stomach. At his age, the weight had become an occupational hazard, making him tired, sluggish, and slow on his feet. "I literally can't afford this weight," he told me. "If I keep gaining, I'll risk not being able to do my job."

Greg was motivated to make changes. He told me that his biggest downfall was dinner. Every night, after a long work shift, he returned home emotionally and physically exhausted. His family life centered on his four-year-old twins, whom he adored but who made his evenings so chaotic that he never had a quiet moment.

Greg's wife, Maria, was a terrific Italian cook. She loved fixing lasagna and ravioli, homemade breads and decadent desserts. Despite reading his advantages list and reminder cards just before he got in the car to drive home, Greg's determination faded by the time he hit the dinner table, and he was unable to eat his dinner slowly and mindfully.

Greg's Advantages List

1. I'll protect my job.
2. I'll have more energy.
3. I'll be healthier in general.
4. I'll reduce my risk of heart disease.
5. I'll be able to move around a lot more easily.
6. I'll be able to play with the kids better.
7. My shirt will stay tucked in.
8. I'll feel better about myself.
9. I'll be able to bend more easily.
10. My body won't feel so heavy.
11. I won't be mad at myself every night.
12. I'll feel proud of myself.

"I just shovel it in," he admitted. "I know I shouldn't. I know that if I enjoy every bite, I probably won't eat as much. But it's just so hard to make myself slow down and think before I eat."

Greg described his routine when he gets home from work. As he walks in the door, his kids, Alma and David, "practically tackle" him. He barely has time to hang up his jacket before his wife calls them to the table. Dinner is noisy. Maria is tired, and she leaves it up to Greg to discipline the twins. He usually tries to ignore the fighting and eat, but it's hard to focus on enjoying the meal or even notice how much he's eaten.

"The kids eat fast," Greg described. "They're done in ten minutes, and then they start pestering us to let them go watch TV."

"And what do you do?"

"I usually tell them they have to stay at the table. But they're hooting and hollering and picking on one another, so finally I tell them they can go. Then I look down at my plate—and my food is usually gone. So I take seconds because I don't feel satisfied." Greg shook his head. "I start off with good intentions but somehow I eat so much more than I meant to. I don't notice half of what I eat. I know I shouldn't have seconds. But I don't feel like I have any willpower."

No wonder—who can appreciate a meal when chaos reigns? First we talked about how Greg could reduce his stress *before* he sat down, so he'd at least set himself up to be able to enjoy his food. Then we did some problem solving about the meal itself. He created a list incorporating many of these ideas.

When I Get Home from Work

1. Sit in my car and listen to relaxing music for at least 5 minutes and then read my advantages list and reminder cards.
2. Ask Maria to have dinner ready 15 minutes after I come in the door so we don't eat right away.
3. When I first get home, hug the kids and read a book to them.
4. While the kids are at the table, eat a salad as slowly as I can and drink a glass of water.
5. Let the twins leave the table when they've finished eating. Then serve myself one plate of food and eat it as slowly and mindfully as possible.
6. If I notice I'm eating too quickly, put down my fork and take a few deep breaths. Don't pick it back up until I can focus on eating again.
7. Ask Maria to leave the serving dishes in the kitchen instead of putting them on the table.

Over the next week, Greg instituted these changes, but he still felt stressed, which made it hard to resist seconds. He asked Maria for advice, and she had a great idea. She suggested that Greg take a quick shower and relax for a few minutes in their bedroom instead of reading a book to the kids. She reminded him that he could read a book to them *after* dinner.

Having this small respite provided Greg with a positive sense of self-nurturing that he'd previously been seeking in food—with no negative consequences! And the nightly ritual of leaving the table to read a book to the kids as soon as he had finished his one plate of food helped him avoid taking seconds.

With this new plan, Greg emerged from his shower refreshed. He felt calmer and had more psychic energy to control his eating. He felt proud of breaking the cycle of overeating that he'd been locked into for years.

Escape the De-Stress with Food Trap

When you don't give yourself enough opportunity to decompress, you run the risk of using food as a pressure valve. Zeroing in on your "hot spots"— your moments of greatest stress—and figuring out how to solve the problem can help you defuse the stress so you don't try to stuff it down with food.

- Identify the problematic situations that contribute to stress.

- Ask a family member or friend to brainstorm solutions with you. Be careful not to prematurely rule any out—your objections might be based on unhelpful sabotaging thoughts.

- Rearrange your activities so you have time to de-stress before meals.

- Create a menu of de-stressing techniques to draw on. Consider, for example, listening to music, taking a bath, sipping a cup of tea, talking to a close friend, going for a walk, meditating, or anything that feels self-nurturing.

#4: The When Things Calm Down Trap

You think it will be too difficult to work on healthy eating during a stressful time.

When she was younger, Kristen had been able to maintain a healthy weight without much effort because of all the sports she played. However, she was now getting older and, as an accountant, had a sedentary desk job. She had been steadily gaining weight each year for at least a decade. After gaining an extra fifty pounds, she realized she couldn't ignore the problem any longer; it was time to work on losing weight.

Kristen was able to move through the initial steps of the program with relative ease, incorporating new habits into her daily life. She was feeling in control and on top of things when a double whammy hit: tax season started, making her hours at work much, much longer; and her husband's small business started having financial problems. Suddenly Kristen's stress levels skyrocketed and she found it much harder to get herself to practice the healthy eating habits that just a few weeks earlier had been no sweat. Some days she was able to get herself to practice her new skills and stay on track, but some days she wasn't. "I think I'm just too stressed to work on dieting right now," she said. "I just have too much to handle."

Sound familiar? You're not alone. Like Kristen, many people think focusing on healthy eating will make a stressful time even more stressful. We have seen over and over, though, that the opposite is invariably true: When you go through a stressful time and lose control over your eating, that loss of control makes you feel *more* stressed. Keeping your eating on track during stressful periods can help you feel generally more in control, *lowering* stress instead of adding to it.

Kristen and I reviewed some of her eating experiences from the past week. She felt proud of passing up a pastry at work. "It was hard to resist," she told me. "They looked really delicious. But as soon as I left the kitchen, I felt really good about not eating any. In fact, I felt good all day that I hadn't given in."

Then I asked her to reflect on how she had felt about overeating at a restaurant the previous night. "I thought eating this big indulgent meal would make me feel better. But it didn't. I just wound up feeling stuffed and mad at myself."

The more she thought about it, the more Kristen realized that resisting the pastry actually reduced her stress. She felt more in control, had more "positive energy," and was better able to focus on her work. On the other hand, overeating at dinner made her feel more stressed because she felt guilty, distracted, and heavier in her body. Then she had a harder time focusing on the work she had brought home.

To help her remember what she had discovered, Kristen made the following reminder card:

> Even though I think maintaining control over my eating will make me feel more stressed, it actually makes me feel less stressed. Remember the pastry! Staying on track, even when it's hard, feels good and reduces my stress.

Escape the When Things Calm Down Trap

When you are busy, you may think you can't possibly be disciplined about eating, too. But exerting your willpower is likely to help you feel better than giving in to your cravings.

- Think about a time when you gave in to a craving and a time when you resisted; which made you feel better an hour later?

- When you're going through a stressful time, take extra care to read your reminder cards often—even several times a day—to help you remember that getting off track with your eating will make you more stressed, not less. (You don't need the additional stress of feeling guilty about something you ate!) Staying on track will help you feel more in control of your eating and more in control in general, which will make you feel less stressed overall.

Creating Escape Plans for Stress Traps

Stress is part of life; there's no chance you're going to be rid of it, so you need to learn how to manage it. Avoiding stress traps requires a multipronged approach. Look for ways to decrease your stress level and increase your self-care. Tune in to your stress eating. Does it truly help you manage stress, or does it make things worse? Then create an escape plan for each difficult situation you identify, using the process described beginning on page 42.

❶ Identify a future situation in which a stress trap might arise.

❷ Predict and record your sabotaging thoughts.

❸ Write a compelling response to each sabotaging thought.

❹ Develop a list of strategies.

❺ Review and revise your escape plan often.

Consider the following sample escape plan as you brainstorm and craft your own.

Escape Plan: Stress Trap

Situation #1: The end of the school year—overwhelmed with year-end activities, recitals, ceremonies, presents, parties. Just don't have the time or energy to keep dieting!

Sabotaging Thoughts	Reminders	Strategies
I can either diet or manage all of my responsibilities, but I can't do both. I can't disappoint the kids by not attending the events they want me to go to. I don't have time to get to the store or exercise. Once school is over and the kids are home for the summer, I'll get back on track with my eating plan.	I will always have stressful times. Losing weight is so important to me that I have to make it a top priority and de-prioritize other things. At this point, it's more important to take care of myself. The kids will get over their disappointment. Besides I can go to some of the events, just not all of them. It will be more difficult to find the time to shop and go to the gym, but it's not impossible. I can't use lack of time as an excuse—not if I truly want to lose weight. This has been my pattern for the past few years and it just doesn't work. I could easily gain back the 5 pounds I just worked so hard to lose. I'll be much happier if I stay on track now.	Look at my schedule for this week and figure out what I can spend less time on or skip altogether. Go to the baseball game late. Ask Rebecca to take the kids to Ben's birthday party. Skip the party for the teachers and staff. Wake up half an hour earlier for the next 2 weeks to get things done. To make sure I get to the market, bring the kids with me after their games instead of dropping them at home. Arrange to pick up Kimi twice this week and go to the gym with her so I won't be tempted to skip it. Read my advantages list and this escape plan 3 times a day until school is over.

Reflect and Recommit:
Why I Want to Escape This Trap

You have a choice. You can keep allowing stress to overwhelm your weight-loss efforts—and suffer the consequences. Or you can decide to make a change. **Stress will be there either way. Do you want to feel stressed and bad about yourself, or do you want to feel stressed and better about yourself?**

Imagine what could happen if you changed unreasonable rules; really prioritized dieting, exercise, and self-care; problem-solved to reduce stress; and reminded yourself that overeating leads to greater stress than staying in control of your eating does.

Commit yourself to working on stress traps right now, so you'll be prepared when the next stressful period arises. Take a few minutes to write one final summary reminder card to motivate you to make changes and keep making changes.

Chapter 4

Emotional Eating Traps

When you hear upsetting news, what is your first instinct? Do you find yourself reaching for sweets?

When you've had a bad day at work, do you stop on the way home to hit the drive-through at a fast-food restaurant or pick up a big bag of chips at a convenience store?

After you've had an argument with a friend, do you head into the kitchen and tear open the bag of chocolate chips you'd been saving to make cookies?

When you experience negative emotions, you may have strong cravings for food. You may even believe that food is the *only* way to calm down. Or you may believe that you deserve to comfort yourself with food when you're upset. Eating becomes your default response to distress. Most people who struggle to lose weight have a habit of turning to food for solace when they feel lonely, worried, angry, or sad.

And in fact, food *can* comfort, console, distract, and soothe. Eating *can* calm you down—but only while you are literally consuming the food and for a very short time afterward. Food will never solve the problem that upset you in the first place. While eating may temporarily distract you from difficult feelings, once that distraction has worn off, you are likely to experience regret for straying from your plan—and you will probably feel even worse than you did before you started eating.

Emotional eating never solves problems. It just creates new ones.

You may also turn to food when you experience minor discomfort. Perhaps you're feeling tired, bored, at loose ends, or you simply want to procrastinate. You may not even be fully aware of how you are feeling but find yourself heading to the kitchen for an unplanned snack.

The way to escape emotional eating traps is to learn how to deal with discomfort in a new way. Instead of turning to food when you experience negative emotions, you can try to solve the problem you're upset about or adopt a more reasonable view of the problem. But if you are seeing the problem accurately and there's nothing you can do at the moment to solve it, you need to learn to accept your distress.

Accepting distress is a learning process. A reasonable interim strategy is to focus on something else. You can begin by distracting yourself with pleasurable or productive activities. When you demonstrate to yourself that you can break the habit of managing negative emotions through eating, you will feel stronger and more in control. As you practice and gain mastery over emotional eating, you will probably experience a tremendous sense of pride and relief that food no longer has power over you.

Let's consider a few of the most common emotional eating traps.

#1: The Trying to Numb Pain Trap

You believe it's not okay to feel negative emotions.

Elizabeth had struggled with her weight for many years, but it wasn't until she was in her sixties that she began to have a serious problem. Things really came to a head when her husband, Bill, who was ten years her senior, began to suffer health problems. Every time he got sick, she became anxious and let her eating "get really out of control."

In fact, *whenever* Elizabeth felt sad, worried, or frustrated, her immediate response was to think about food: *I need to eat something to calm down.* And the food she turned to wasn't of the healthy variety. She ate sweets—lots of them. She believed that experiencing negative emotion was "bad" and that she needed to eat to get rid of her uncomfortable feelings.

First we talked about what might happen if Elizabeth *didn't* eat when she was distressed. Elizabeth said she thought she'd feel increasingly upset until she finally couldn't tolerate the feeling any longer.

I asked Elizabeth to think of recent times when she felt significant distress but didn't eat. The first experience she told me about had occurred the previous month. She had accompanied Bill to his doctor's appointment, where they were told he needed an operation. "I was really upset," she said, "but I couldn't eat. I wanted to but I didn't have the opportunity. By the time we left the doctor's office, it was almost lunchtime. But first we had to go to the lab so he could get some blood work done, which took forever. Then when we finally left, our car had a flat tire and AAA took over an hour to get to us. Then we had to stop at a second pharmacy for Bill's medicine because the first one was out of what he needed. When we finally got home, it was almost dinnertime."

"And what had you eaten since you left the doctor's office?"

"Nothing," Elizabeth replied.

She had a perfect example of an experience when she was very upset but didn't eat. She had gotten through it. And how would she have felt if she had had access to junk food and had eaten it all afternoon?

"Bad," she said. "I mean, I would have excused myself some, but I know it's unhealthy for me." She captured that experience on a reminder card so she could remember that she didn't need to self-medicate with food to get through a trying experience:

I was really upset after the appointment with Dr. Ross, but I got through the whole rest of the afternoon without eating. This shows it's not true that I need to eat when I'm upset. I may want to eat, but I don't need to eat.

Next we talked about how emotions aren't inherently good or bad. Emotions are simply part of our human experience. In fact, negative emotions can serve an important function, alerting us to a problem that may need our attention. To break the cycle of emotional eating, we need to accept all our emotions, not just the positive ones.

To help Elizabeth recognize that intense emotions have peaks and troughs, I asked her to visualize a negative emotion as a big wave in the ocean. Like a wave, emotional pain can build up and become more intense, but it always crests, and then starts to come down, even if you don't do anything to make it go away. Elizabeth made a reminder card for these ideas:

> When I was the most upset I ever remember feeling, I still survived. Negative emotions aren't bad. They are part of being human. I don't need to make them go away. Negative emotions always crest, like a wave, and then start to come down. I don't have to be afraid of my feelings.

Escape the Trying to Numb Pain Trap

Many emotional eating traps share a bit in common with this trap. At its root, this trap is about numbing pain. But if you think back over your history, you will likely find plenty of evidence that you *can* tolerate negative feelings. You are undoubtedly stronger than you think; you don't need food to manage upsetting emotions. You just think you do. To develop trust in your ability to handle difficult feelings, you need to stop using food to decrease your distress.

- Think about the most distressed you've ever been. Call that a ten on a ten-point scale. Then do an experiment. The next time you're upset, set a timer for twenty minutes. Don't do anything to try to reduce your negative emotion. Don't fight it. Just measure it on your ten-point scale. See what happens when you experience negative emotions and just accept feeling that way.

- Reflect on past experiences of emotional distress when you weren't able to turn to food to feel better. How intense did the distress get? How long did it last at that peak level? Did it continue to go up and up until a catastrophe happened? Or did it rise, crest, and fall; then rise, crest, and fall again?

#2: The No Alternatives Trap

You believe that if you're upset, the only thing you can do is eat.

As Elizabeth's husband continued to experience health problems, developing alternative coping skills became increasingly important. Now that she knew negative emotions weren't harmful, we were able to talk about strategies that would be healthier and more helpful than turning to food.

I asked Elizabeth whether she knew other people who didn't turn to food when they were upset. "Well, yes," she said. Her husband turned out to be a great example. His eating remained pretty much the same from day to day. When Bill was upset about his medical condition, for example, he didn't turn to food. Instead, he talked to Elizabeth, took a short walk, or distracted himself by reading.

Elizabeth's husband was a good role model for coping with negative emotion. "I guess I've just always used food as a coping strategy," she told me. "When I was a kid, my grandmother used to give me cookies whenever my older brother was really mean to me," she said. "I think ever since then I've associated feeling bad with eating."

Even if you have had a long history of calming yourself with food, it doesn't mean you can't change. Eating to soothe upsetting emotions is a

learned behavior that you can *unlearn*. Elizabeth made a reminder card
to help her remember this idea:

> I learned to eat when I was feeling bad, but now I can unlearn it. Bill doesn't eat when he's upset. It's not a given that food is the only way to feel better.

The following week, Elizabeth asked a couple of close friends and her
sister what they did when they were upset. She was full of interesting
information at our next session.

"It was really an eye-opener," Elizabeth said, as she pulled out her
notes. "My sister said she tries to solve the problem, and if she can't, she
focuses on getting things done around the house. My neighbor Isabella
just tries to distract herself. My friend Tracy does deep breathing and
meditation or yoga."

I asked Elizabeth to consider which of these strategies might work
for her. "I guess I eat when I'm upset to distract myself from the problem, so distractions might help. I usually find it hard to focus on solving a problem when I'm upset, so I think it's better to try to calm down
first."

Elizabeth and I made a list of distractions she could try the next time
she was distressed. Watching television or reading a book hadn't diverted
her attention enough in the past, so we left those off the list. Instead, we
tried to think of activities that would be truly absorbing. After some discussion, Elizabeth made the following list.

Distracting Activities

When I'm upset, try one of these distractions. If I still feel the urge to eat, try others until the urge to eat goes away.

1. Call a friend (Alice, Robin, or Neil).
2. Write an e-mail to someone I haven't connected with in a while (Rob, Jonah).
3. Clean out a drawer in the kitchen.
4. Drink hot tea and watch the birds outside.
5. Listen to classical music.
6. Read the newspaper headlines until I find an article that interests me.
7. Play a word game on the iPad.
8. Accept feeling upset without trying to distract myself.

Just reading through this list seemed to calm Elizabeth. She said she would continue to add to the list as she thought of other distracting activities.

A secondary problem with believing that if you're upset the only thing you can do is eat occurs *after* you eat: the inevitable consequences. Elizabeth and I talked about the numerous problems that arise after she uses food to soothe herself. She wrote down the gist of our discussion:

If I eat when I'm upset, I'll only feel momentary comfort. Then I'll have 3 problems: the original problem, then feeling bad and out of control, and then gaining weight. When I want to eat for emotional reasons, ask myself whether I want 1 problem or 3 problems.

Escape the No Alternatives Trap

To escape this trap, you will need to test the idea that eating is the only way you can calm down. In actuality, you just have a strong habit of eating when you're upset. You may continue to rely on food until you develop confidence that you can handle negative emotions. In the meantime, distraction can help you avoid eating.

- Think of as many examples as you can of occasions when you felt upset but had no access to food. What did you do? Did you eventually calm down? How accurate is it to say that you have to eat to calm down? Write a reminder card to reinforce the idea that the only way to decrease negative emotion is through food.

- Make a list of activities you can engage in instead of eating—for instance, people to call or e-mail, websites to visit, videos to watch, errands to run. There's also music, meditation, exercise, crafts or hobbies, yard work, housework, a soothing bath or cup of tea—so many possibilities. But don't wait until you're in distress to make this list or you'll likely just end up eating.

- For additional ideas, ask a friend. Or enter "pleasurable activities" in a search engine.

- Once you have your list, see which activities require advance preparation. Do you need to buy a book of crossword puzzles? Inflate the tires on your bike so you can take a ride? Put any required objects (your scrapbook, magazines) along with a copy of the list in an easily accessible box so everything will be ready and waiting when you're upset and have the urge to eat.

#3: The Entitlement Eating Trap

You believe you deserve to comfort yourself with food.

Sometimes emotional eating traps take a slightly different form: you may or may not believe that you *have* to eat to feel better, but you think you are *entitled* to eat.

Beth, a social worker, took care of many people at work but did not always do a great job of taking care of herself. Many evenings she left work upset, still thinking about a problem one of her clients was facing. Then she'd stop at a fast-food restaurant, get a really big meal at the drive-through, and finish it while she was driving home. Although Beth knew that eating fast food had packed on the pounds, she found she was unable to stop herself; those meals felt nurturing. She had spent all day trying to help others feel better. "Eating feels like what I do to take care of myself, to make *me* feel better," she explained.

I questioned whether those fast-food meals actually did make her feel better.

"Well, yes," she replied. "It's my treat." Then she paused. "I do feel better while I'm eating, but . . ." Her voice trailed off.

"But?"

"But I have to admit, I feel bad afterward. I feel overstuffed, weak, . . . and guilty. I know how bad fast food is for me. I'm embarrassed. I would hate it if anyone saw me eating it."

And what impact did it have on reaching her goal of losing weight?

"Well, it's making it nearly impossible," Beth said. "Even if I've been really good during the day, fast food has so many calories. I know I can't keep doing it and lose weight. But I keep thinking, 'I had such a hard day. Aren't I entitled to feel better?'"

"Of course you are!" I exclaimed. "But aren't you also entitled to get all the benefits of losing weight?" She nodded and gave me a half smile. "Then we just need to figure out how you can feel better without eating." She made a reminder card to remember this idea:

When I want to eat fast food after an upsetting day at work, remember: I'm entitled to take care of myself and I'm entitled to feel better, but I'm also entitled to get everything on my advantages list, so I have to find other ways to comfort myself. (Besides, eating it always makes me feel worse afterward.)

Beth needed strategies to help her get over her fast-food habit. After a bit of discussion, she decided she would spend time on Sundays cooking for the week so she'd have a healthy meal waiting for her at home every night. Then she'd be less likely to stop at a fast-food place after work.

"If you had a hard day at work and came home and ate a delicious, healthy meal, how do you think you would feel?" I asked.

"Well, I'm not sure it would make me feel better, but I'm sure it wouldn't make me feel worse."

"Let me ask you another question. How do you think you'll feel if you leave work, eat a delicious, healthy meal, start to lose weight, and begin to get the advantages on your list: feeling better about yourself, fitting into your clothes, being able to exercise more easily, having more self-confidence socially, and things like that?"

"I'll definitely feel good!"

Beth made a reminder card to read right before she left work:

> Even if I had a hard day, go straight home and eat the healthy meal that's waiting for me. Doing that will make me feel good and I'll feel great when I lose weight. Stopping to get unhealthy fast food will just make me feel terrible.

Next we did some problem solving in case she didn't have time to prepare a meal or ran out of healthy food. She came up with ideas for some quick and healthy options she could get on the way home from work. She made a list of restaurants and food shops and jotted down specific items she would get.

Then I asked her whether getting unhealthy fast food *was* really a treat, given how she felt afterward. She created another reminder card:

Fast food may seem like a treat, but it's actually the opposite of a treat when I impulsively get unhealthy food and overeat. I should occasionally plan in advance to get a fast-food meal, bring it home, eat it slowly, and enjoy every bite. In between, if I want to treat myself, I should do it in nonfood ways. I could get a new book, a nice-smelling candle, a new nail polish color, or a celebrity magazine.

We also started a list of self-soothing activities Beth could do when she needed comfort. She added to the list in the coming weeks.

Comforting Activities

- Take a hot bath with aromatherapy.

- Turn on loud music and dance.

- Curl up on the sofa with a blanket and watch a romantic comedy.

- Look at my favorite pictures of friends and family.

- Walk Max, groom him, or cuddle with him on the sofa.

With these strategies in place, Beth was finally able to overcome the habit of soothing herself with food. The first few weeks were difficult; she still had to fight against her "giving-in" muscle's strong urge to stop at a fast-food restaurant. But as time went on, her resistance muscle became stronger, and resisting became easier and easier. She gradually had less and less trouble going straight home, eating a healthy dinner, and remembering to consult her ever-growing list of self-soothing activities, which helped her get the comfort she was entitled to. She felt better *and* she lost weight.

Escape the Entitlement Eating Trap

People often get tripped up by their concept of being entitled to feel better. Of course they're entitled to feel better! But trying to feel better through overeating backfires. It's simply incompatible with the goal of losing weight and keeping it off. Like Elizabeth, you have to decide: either continue to overeat and feel better *temporarily* (and worse soon after) *or* comfort yourself in nonfood ways, lose weight, and start reaping the rewards. To escape this trap:

- Read your advantages list often. You might even create multiple sets of cards, using creative lettering, different colors, photos, or images. The act of writing and routinely repeating these ideas to yourself will carve those neural grooves a little deeper.

- Ask yourself which entitlement you want more: delaying distress for a few minutes or getting the advantages of healthy eating and weight loss? Consider posting a copy of your advantages list in your most vulnerable areas, such as the fridge or the pantry door.

- Create your own list of comforting activities, and continue adding to it as you think of new ideas. Look for boards on Pinterest, or follow pages on Facebook or Instagram that post clever ideas for pleasurable activities.

#4: The Killing Time Trap

You turn to food when you're bored, tired, or procrastinating.

Beth still struggled to control her eating in the evening. Some nights she would find herself, around nine or ten, standing in front of the refrigerator just wanting to eat *anything*. I asked Beth to think about where she felt the desire to eat. Was it in her stomach? Did she have an empty sensation in her abdomen? Or was she experiencing sensations elsewhere in her body—in her mouth, throat, upper body? Beth wasn't sure, so she agreed to monitor herself over the coming week. She would gauge how she felt just before she went to the refrigerator, and she'd be on the lookout for where in her body the desire to eat was coming from.

Over the next week, Beth gathered some interesting data. On evenings when she was tempted to overeat, she found she was either feeling bored (with nothing she really felt like doing) or she was procrastinating (because there was something she *should* be doing but didn't want to), or she was tired (but didn't feel like going to bed). She also realized that during these evening visits to the refrigerator, she didn't have an empty sensation in her stomach.

Even though she labeled what she was feeling as hunger, she wasn't actually experiencing symptoms of hunger. And no wonder—she had usually just finished eating a substantial dinner an hour or two before. "I hadn't realized it, but the desire to eat was coming from my mouth," she said. "That surprised me. I guess it wasn't hunger. I just *wanted* to eat." She made a reminder card about this:

> If I feel like eating in the evening, remind myself that I'm probably just at loose ends, not hungry, so eating isn't the answer. Find something else to do. If I eat, I'll reinforce my giving-in habit, feel bad about myself, and stay overweight, and I don't want that.

Beth realized that she often had the desire to eat while watching television at night, especially when the program was somewhat boring. She channel surfed but often couldn't find anything that really interested her. We talked about some options:

- She could stop watching television and find a more engaging activity.

- She could find something else to do besides eating while she watched television.

- She could watch television and just accept the mildly bored feeling.

Beth weighed her options and decided she'd like to have a number of activities to choose from. First we talked about what she could do *while* watching television. "I'd like to get back to knitting," she said. "I had been working on this sweater but I got too busy a few months ago and put it away." Then we discussed a few other possibilities, and Beth made a list.

When I'm Bored (Instead of or While Watching TV)

1. Knit and listen to music.

2. Check out Facebook or YouTube.

3. Plan a vacation.

4. Do Sudoku or crossword puzzles.

5. Make an online dating profile and start to look at what guys have posted.

6. Call Thea or Jody.

Beth also recognized that feeling tired in the evening sometimes drove her to eat. "I feel kind of logy a lot of times at night. Eating wakes me up a little so I can do things, like finish chores." She agreed that doing ten jumping jacks might serve the same purpose. At other times, Beth ate because she didn't feel like getting ready for bed and eating let her postpone the inevitable. I explained that eating when tired led to weight gain. And going to bed later than she should made her more tired the next day—which made it harder to stick to her plan.

To steer herself away from tired eating, Beth instituted a mandatory bedtime: in bed by ten-thirty and lights out by eleven. She set two alarms on her phone:

- The first would go off at ten-fifteen, as a reminder that she had fifteen minutes to wrap up whatever she was doing.

- The second would go off at ten-thirty, to remind her that it was time to get in bed.

And she made the following reminder card:

Nothing good ever happens when I stay up past 11. I just eat (actually overeat) to stay awake, and then I feel tired and stressed the next day. Get in bed. Anything I'm doing will still be there tomorrow.

Finally we discussed eating as a form of procrastination, such as when she had to pay bills or fill out health insurance forms. We talked about how she could spend just five minutes on a task she felt like avoiding and then decide whether to continue it or start another noneating activity. Or she could decide to avoid the task but commit to a specific time to do it within the next few days.

Beth worked hard in the coming few weeks to label what she was experiencing when she wanted to eat but wasn't hungry and to learn to accept feeling the mild—and temporary—discomfort of not eating after her planned snack at night. She realized that the greater discomfort of being overweight would go on and on if she kept eating. Staying in control of her eating got progressively easier the more she told herself, "I'm just bored (or tired or feel like procrastinating). That's not a reason to eat. Go do something else. This feeling will pass." And it always did.

Escape the Killing Time Trap

Many dieters don't recognize their eating triggers, especially if the trigger is mild discomfort. The next time you find yourself eating and aren't sure why, ask yourself whether you're feeling a little uncomfortable or fatigued. If so, you will need to break the cycle.

- When you're tempted to eat even though you haven't been triggered by hunger or specific foods, ask yourself whether you're bored, at loose ends, or procrastinating. Label the feeling. Just the awareness alone is sometimes enough to break the spell.

- Create a reminder card so you will remember the consequences of unplanned eating.

- If you eat to improve alertness, try some quick exercise instead.

- Ask yourself if you'd rather stay overweight or break the habit of eating when you're not supposed to. Create a list of other activities to refocus your attention away from food or choose to accept the mild discomfort you're experiencing.

Creating Escape Plans for Emotional Eating

We have found that most people who struggle with dieting stumble into emotional eating traps because they have entrenched habits of using food to make themselves feel better. But the consequences of using eating as a coping strategy can bring huge, long-lasting disadvantages. Consider whether any of the emotional eating traps apply to you, then create your own escape plans.

❶ **Identify a future situation in which an emotional eating trap might arise.**

❷ **Record your sabotaging thoughts.**

❸ **Write a compelling response to each sabotaging thought.**

❹ **Develop a list of strategies.**

❺ **Review and revise your escape plan often.**

Consider the following sample escape plan as you brainstorm and craft your own.

Escape Plan: Emotional Eating Trap

Situation #1: Feeling lonely at night. I'm sad that my husband and I have grown apart. Sometimes it seems like food is my best friend.

Sabotaging Thoughts	Reminders	Strategies
I'm lonely. I deserve to treat myself with extra ice cream. Ice cream is the only thing that makes me feel better. It's not fair that I can't comfort myself with food.	It's true that I'm lonely. I need to accept the feeling and deal with loneliness in another way. If I binge on ice cream, I'll still feel lonely plus I'll feel bad about myself. It's not true that ice cream is the only thing that makes me feel better. I'd also feel better if I called my friends and connected with them. What would be even more unfair is if I let a sense of unfairness stand in my way of losing weight, which is really important to me.	Start buying only a single ice cream treat each day to eat at night. Throw away the pints of ice cream that are already in the freezer. Figure out ways to get together with friends on at least a couple of evenings a week. Go to the movies by myself. Save errands for nighttime. Call Ruthie! Call Maureen! Connect with Lois and Barbara through e-mail. Ask Phyllis to take a walk with me after dinner on weekdays. Look into taking a Spanish course. Enlist my friends to help me figure out what else to do to make my life better.

Reflect and Recommit: Why I Want to Escape This Trap

Emotional eating is a learned behavior, and it is entirely optional. You can make the choice to allow emotional eating to control you and derail your weight-loss efforts. Or you can make a change.

When you're upset, would you rather have just the original problem that distressed you? Or do you want to have that problem plus feeling bad about overeating? And then add the problem of extra pounds as well?

In other words, do you want to have one problem—or do you want to have three?

Emotional eating traps require a consistent, steady response, and those habits can be hard to kick. The more you can predict upsetting situations, the more you can prepare yourself to do something other than eating. Start right now, so you'll be ready when the next wave of negative feelings washes over you. Take a few minutes to write one final summary reminder card to motivate you to make changes and keep making changes.

PART THREE

Interpersonal Traps: How Others Trap Me

Chapter 5

Food Pusher Traps

Almost every dieter who tries to lose weight is going to face food pushers at one time or another. Some food pushers can be easily put off by a "No, thank you" or two. Others are more insistent. Some food pushers want you to eat the food they're pushing on you because they genuinely want you to experience the flavor or appreciate their efforts; others believe it's polite or expected to insist. Some may even push food on you because they're actively trying to sabotage your diet.

Regardless of who the food pushers are or the motives behind the pushing, your ability to stand firm and say no is always under your control—once you learn how to challenge sabotaging thoughts. In this chapter, we'll talk about how you can escape from food pusher traps; some of these concepts will play out even more dramatically in chapter 6, "Family Traps."

#1: The Chronic Hard Sell Trap

People keep pushing you to eat even when you say no.

Raised in a big family, Laura was the middle child of five siblings and often found herself in the role of peacemaker. Loud voices and confrontations always made her uncomfortable, and as she grew older, this desire to avoid conflict grew stronger. Now in her early thirties, Laura often found it difficult to stand up for herself or say no to people—particularly her siblings.

When Laura first came to see me one spring day, she told me she had wanted to get help with dieting for a long time. She was a classic yo-yo dieter, always losing and then gaining back the same ten pounds, which really showed on her petite frame. Laura quickly mastered the foundation strategies because she was usually able to stick to a plan during the year. But summer was fast approaching, when staying on track would be most difficult for her.

Some people find summer the easiest season to lose weight, because dishes are usually lighter and we have more opportunities to be active outside. But for Laura, summer was the total opposite. Her parents owned a place in the mountains, and each summer, the entire family descended on the cottage every weekend they could.

"It's usually a lot of fun," Laura said. "We swim in the lake, hike a lot, we cook together. But in terms of my eating, it's really, really hard." She would follow her food plan all winter and spring and feel good about herself when summer began. But her healthy eating habits fell by the wayside on the free-for-all weekends. Everyone ate and drank pretty much without restraint and pushed Laura to do the same. No matter how much she tried to resist, it didn't help. "I always end up giving in," she sighed. "It's really frustrating. By the end of the summer, I gain back whatever I had lost during the rest of the year, and I have to start all over again. I'm in a bad cycle, and I want to change it."

First we needed to figure out what type of food pushers she was dealing with. "When your family pushes food and drinks on you, do you think they're doing it so you'll be taking part in the things they're doing?" I asked. "Or are they deliberately trying to sabotage you?"

Laura said they definitely fell in the first category. "I guess they think I won't have fun—or maybe they think *they* won't have as much fun—if I don't eat and drink like them," she said. Laura described a typical Saturday night. The family would have a big barbecue on the deck, with lots of beer and the works: hamburgers, hot dogs, ribs, corn on the cob, coleslaw, and potato salad. And at least a couple of desserts.

I asked Laura to describe a specific incident that exemplified the problem. She remembered an occasion when she had decided to limit herself to one hamburger and one beer so she could eat the side dishes she really liked and a piece of chocolate cake (with really good icing) from her favorite bakery. But the moment Laura's older sister, Sharon, saw her refuse a second beer, the drink pushing started.

"Come on, have another beer," Sharon had said. Laura declined, but Sharon kept pushing. "Come on, what's the big deal? You always have more than one. It's our family tradition!" And on and on until, wanting to avoid conflict, Laura finally gave in and took another beer. And another one after that. She was concerned that history would repeat itself this summer.

"We have a big barbecue coming up next weekend," Laura said, "and my whole family will be there because it's the first weekend of the season." She wanted to stick to the eating plan she'd made last summer. But she was afraid a family member would insist that she eat or drink something she hadn't planned. She looked down. "I really don't want a repeat of all the other weekends at the lake."

I suggested to Laura that we role-play to help her learn what to do. I played Laura, and she played Sharon. She started.

"Laura, have another beer."

"No, thanks."

"Oh, Laura, not *this* again! It's just one beer!"

"No, thanks."

"Oh, come on. Join the fun! You never have just one."

"No, thank you."

"What's the problem?"

"No problem. And no, thanks."

"But it's more fun when you drink."

"No, thank you."

"But it's our family tradition! You don't want to break tradition, do you?"

"No, thank you."

"You know you'll end up drinking more later anyway."

"No, thank you."

"You're really not having another one?"

"No thanks."

"Really?"

"No, thanks."

Laura and I discussed the role play and my use of the "broken-record" technique—not offering reasons but instead just saying, "No, thank you," whenever food or drink was pushed. "What did you think?" I asked her.

"That was good," she replied. "I eventually couldn't think of any other ways to push, and I gave up." I asked Laura if she thought Sharon would eventually give up, too. She did but then expressed another concern. "I think she'd then go complain to my other sister that I wasn't drinking." Laura didn't like the idea of her sisters talking about her.

The anticipation of feeling uncomfortable when food pushers complain to others can really be a deterrent. To counter this, it's important for you to recognize the payoffs of standing firm and to realize that you can cope with feeling uncomfortable.

I referred to the advantages list Laura had made back in our first session and asked her about the disadvantages she would face if she gained weight, then questioned which scenario would make her feel more uncomfortable:

- having her sisters talk about her not having a beer; or

- constantly giving in, starting the cycle of eating and drinking too much, feeling guilty and out of control, feeling frustrated with herself and the food pushers, undoing her hard work of healthy eating during the rest of the year, having to wear clothes that grew progressively tighter as the summer went on, and feeling self-conscious at the lake.

"It's no contest," she concluded. "Gaining weight again this summer would be *so* much more uncomfortable, for so much longer." Laura realized that either way she was going to feel uncomfortable. She would either have to deal with the *momentary* and *mild* discomfort of having her sisters talk about her or the greater and longer-lasting discomfort of gaining weight. Laura made the following reminder card to help her remember both how and why she would stick to her guns:

> When my family pushes food on me, just keep saying, "No, thanks." Eventually they'll run out of things to say and give up. JUST SAY NO!!! If they complain about me, I'll feel momentary discomfort, but if I don't stick up for myself, I'll feel much more uncomfortable and for much, much longer.

Escape the Chronic Hard Sell Trap

In some ways, the best tactic to counter the chronic hard sell is just endurance—as long as your food pusher has no malicious intent, simple repetition of the words *no, thanks* can work wonders. After demonstrating to food pushers on several occasions that you won't be pushed around, they usually learn that you're not going to give in and stop pushing.

- To overcome food pushers, try the "broken-record" technique. Keep saying, "No, thank you," over and over again to whatever they say.

- You never need to give a reason for why you're turning down food or drink. You can offer one, though, if you want. Here are some variations you can try:

"Thanks, I don't want any."

"I've already had some."

"I may have some later."

"I'm not hungry."

"I couldn't fit in another bite, but thank you."

- Saying no to food pushers can be uncomfortable—but so is giving in! Ask yourself, Which discomfort would I rather experience? The momentary discomfort of saying no or the much more far-reaching discomfort of giving in and sabotaging my efforts to lose weight?

#2: The Passive Pushee Trap

You wait for the pusher to stop pushing rather than just refusing.

We often hear dieters grumble about food pushers, "It's so annoying. Why won't my friend just stop pestering me to eat something?" or "It's so unfair that my cousin keeps insisting that I have seconds even when I say I don't want any more." These dieters are making the classic mistake of expecting the food pusher to be the one to change when, in fact, the initial change needs to come from dieters themselves. Laura, too, was struggling with this notion.

"It's just so hard to deal with my family sometimes!" she exclaimed. "I wish they would just stop trying to get me to eat more than I want."

"It's true. It is hard," I empathized. "But let me ask you something. In the past, what has happened when your family has pushed food on you?"

"I almost always end up giving in," she sighed.

"Exactly!"

Laura had inadvertently taught her family to keep pushing because when they do, they get what they want. No wonder they keep pushing! I helped Laura see that it's not her family's responsibility to stop pushing food on her. "They're food pushers; that's what they do," I said lightly. "It's *your* responsibility to stop saying okay. The first change has to come from you, not from them."

Laura had never thought about the situation in this way. Like many other dieters, she was hoping for the day when her food pushers would just stop pushing her around so she wouldn't have to keep saying no. But the more dieters give in, the more likely their friends and family are to push food on them in the future. Laura found this concept helpful. She made a reminder card:

It's not my family's job to stop pushing food on me. They're food pushers; that's what they do. It is my job to stop giving in. I have to be the one to change.

Escape the Passive Pushee Trap

When food pushers are skilled in the art of pushing food, they can be persistent and tough. Like any skill, being assertive with them takes practice. But what a great payoff when they learn that you're no longer a pushover! You're not going to eat and drink just because they tell you to.

- If you feel frustrated by food pushers, remember that they're just fulfilling their roles. It's *not* their job to take the first step in changing; it's yours. Many dieters find that once they view the trap this way, they find it much easier to overcome.

- If you want food pushers to stop, you have to prove to them that pushing is futile. The more you give in, the more you demonstrate to them that they'll get their way if they just continue to insist. Once you make the decision to stick up for yourself, do it every time or the process of training the food pusher to stop will take much longer.

#3: The Buzz Kill Trap

You feel responsible for making other people feel better about what they're eating and drinking.

Laura had another difficulty with her family food pushers. "I always feel guilty when I say no to drinks they push on me," she said. "I don't want to make them feel bad about how much *they're* drinking."

I had another reality check for her: while it *was* Laura's responsibility to start saying no to food pushers, it *wasn't* Laura's responsibility to make other people feel good about *their* food and drink choices. The bottom line for any of us is that we're only responsible for our own choices; we're not responsible for the choices other people make.

Laura realized that being more concerned about her family's emotional comfort than her own had led her to feel bad about her own eating and drinking—and to end up many pounds heavier than she wanted to be. Just as it was a new idea for Laura that the burden to say no to food pushers fell on her, not her family, it was a revelation for Laura that she didn't have to eat or drink to make others happy. Laura had functioned for so long in the role of peacemaker that she had truly lost sight of the necessity of making decisions that were good for her, not good for everyone *but* her.

"And you know what?" she said. "I usually don't enjoy the stupid beer or food because I'm feeling frustrated that they pushed it on me!"

Laura made the following reminder card:

It's __not__ my responsibility to make my family feel good about what they eat and drink, but it __is__ my responsibility to make healthy choices that make me feel good. When I give in to a food pusher, I don't much enjoy the extra food or drink anyway because I feel upset with myself and them.

Laura looked jubilant when she arrived at my office the next week. "I did it!" she burst out. "This weekend went so much better than any time last summer." Although it had been difficult, Laura had worked hard on saying no to her family. She found that having a written plan of what she intended to eat and drink and reading her reminder cards and advantages list several times a day had really helped her stick to her guns.

At the Saturday night barbecue, her youngest brother kept offering her extra food: "Are you sure you don't want more corn or a hot dog? If you don't eat them, they'll just go to waste. What happened to you? Did you lose your appetite somewhere?"

But Laura just kept declining and then changed the subject. "Hey, how are the repairs going for the sailboat? Can we go out on the lake with it next weekend?"

A few minutes later, Sharon started in when Laura turned down a second beer, but Laura persevered. She steadfastly and persistently said no four times. As predicted, her beer-pushing sister then walked right over to their younger sister, Eliza, to complain about Laura. Although Laura felt uncomfortable, she kept reminding herself that this was easier to deal with than the discomfort of gaining weight. "And you know what? After a little while, she shut up about it, and the night went on and I felt really, really good."

Laura made the following entry in the "worth-it memories" section of her notebook.

May 30

I'm so proud of myself. For the first time, I turned down extra food and beer at the family barbecue! I was just really persistent in saying "no, thanks" and it worked. When I told Sharon I didn't want another beer, she pushed and pushed, but I stuck to my guns. I finally stood up to her! When she complained about me to Eliza, I felt uncomfortable but it wasn't that bad. I could deal with it, and pretty soon they stopped talking about it. I was so glad I didn't give in. It was absolutely 100% worth it to say no.

I told Laura that this summer would probably be the hardest one. "Imagine if you had known how to say no every weekend last summer. What would your family have learned about you?" Laura realized that by now her family would already be used to her new behavior. They would know that "Laura doesn't drink more than one beer. Laura turns down seconds." She could look forward to this scenario next year if she continued to stand up for herself this summer. Laura wanted to remember this point:

> *The next few weekends will be the hardest to say no to my family. Once they get used to the new me, they won't bother me as much to eat and drink the way they do. I have to stick to my guns and prove to them I won't back down and they'll adjust. And besides, being assertive wasn't as hard as I thought it would be.*

When the summer was over, Laura told me that learning to stand firm with her food pushers had helped her learn to stick up more for her own needs in general. "I'm starting to notice other ways I give in to other people, and not just my family, when I shouldn't." What a growth experience the summer had provided!

Escape the Buzz Kill Trap

The realization that you are not responsible for other people's reactions—as long as you're being reasonable—can be a watershed moment that affects not only your ability to stick to a healthy eating plan but can also apply to other important areas of your life. If you feel responsible for making other people feel better about what they eat and drink, remember that when it comes to eating (and your health and sense of well-being), your first responsibility is to yourself.

- Resolve to make eating decisions on the basis of what's important to you, not to others. Watch out for putting other people's feelings above your own. If they feel bad about their own eating behavior, it's not your responsibility.

- Establish a "new normal" with food pushers. As with all new things, the first few times will be the hardest. Stick to your guns and demonstrate to them that you never give in.

- Are there other areas in your life where you are taking excessive responsibility for other people's reactions? How else might your life improve if you started consistently sticking up for yourself (for example, saying no to unreasonable requests, arranging get-togethers when it's convenient for you)?

#4: The People Pleaser Trap

You're concerned you'll disappoint food pushers by turning down their food.

Theresa had been moderately overweight ever since she was a young child. But she had gained an additional thirty pounds in the five years since she had started teaching. She was feeling out of control. If she didn't do something, her weight would most likely keep going up, a prospect that alarmed her. Theresa and her husband were planning to start a family in the next couple of years, and she wanted to be as healthy as possible before she got pregnant.

Theresa initially had difficulty with some of the foundation strategies, but she kept plugging away. She found she was able to control her eating during the work week, but weekends were another story.

Weekends are difficult for many people. Your time is usually less structured, you tend to socialize more, and sabotaging thoughts may give you permission to loosen up. Unfortunately, a few indulgent meals or extra snacks or drinks can lead to gaining back whatever weight you had lost during the week. Unstructured eating on the weekend can also wreak havoc with your resistance muscle, your sense of self-control, and your self-confidence.

Every Sunday, Theresa and her husband have lunch with her mother-in-law, Suzanne, who is a good cook. Theresa described her experience of the previous Sunday. She was able to maintain control and eat reasonable portions, but she got into trouble after lunch, when Suzanne served a great-looking fruit tart. When Suzanne offered her a slice, Theresa politely turned her down. But Suzanne kept pushing, and Theresa ultimately gave in.

"Afterward I felt guilty . . . and weak. We went home, and I just gave up," Theresa said. "I wasn't even hungry, but I kept eating chips and popcorn and a lot of other stuff. I just couldn't seem to get myself back on track until the next day. I want to learn how to stand up to her, but it'll be hard," she said. "I don't want to disappoint her."

I asked Theresa some questions:

- "What other disappointments has Suzanne experienced in her life? Was she able to weather those?"

- "If you turn down her dessert, how strong will her disappointment be? How long will it last?"

- "Will there be any other costs to Suzanne?"

Theresa surmised that Suzanne's disappointment would likely be mild and fleeting, especially compared to the disappointment her mother-in-law had felt when she'd been turned down for a promotion at work. She couldn't think of any other costs to Suzanne if she held her ground.

Now it was time to identify the consequences *Theresa* would face if she gave in to her food-pushing mother-in-law.

- "What are the costs to you if you say yes?"

- "How disappointed will *you* be if you eat off track for the rest of the day and undo your hard work from the past week? How disappointed will you be if you continue this pattern and don't lose weight? How long will *your* disappointment last?"

- "What other costs will there be to you?"

As Theresa answered these questions, I made a cost analysis chart so she could see the consequences in black and white.

Cost to Suzanne if I turn down dessert	Costs to me if I give in to her food pushing
Mild, brief disappointment	Eating extra food and gaining weight
	Feeling weak and guilty for giving in
	Feeling a loss of control over my eating
	Greatly increasing the likelihood of overeating later on
	Strengthening my giving-in muscle
	Continuing an unhealthy pattern
	Feeling very disappointed for a long time when I keep gaining whatever weight I've lost

Seeing the consequences in black and white made the choice stark. Theresa made herself a reminder card to read every day that week in preparation for the following Sunday:

Remember the cost analysis. When I turn down dessert at Suzanne's, she may be a little disappointed for a little while, but she'll get over it. If I give in, I'll have many, many negative consequences. It's worth it to stand firm.

Escape the People Pleaser Trap

Sometimes we unduly focus on and magnify the cost to the food pusher if we resist. We just don't recognize the consequences when we let a food pusher hold sway over us.

- Do a cost analysis: What are the costs to the food pusher if you say no? How great are the consequences to him/her? How long will they last?

- Consider the costs to you if you give in. How great are the consequences to you? How long will they last?

- Think about what advice you'd give to a friend if the costs to him or her of a certain decision were much more severe than the costs to another person.

#5: The Illegitimate to Say No Trap

You feel it's not legitimate to say no to food pushers.

I wanted to find out whether anything else might interfere with Theresa's ability to resist her mother-in-law's food pushing: "How likely are you to say no when she offers you dessert this coming Sunday?"

"Pretty likely," she said, a bit hesitantly.

"What might go through your mind?" I asked.

"I don't know. I guess I usually think about how she really wants me to eat the dessert she baked. We're at her place, she's gone to a lot of trouble . . ." Theresa's voice trailed off.

Like many dieters, Theresa believed her desire to lose weight wasn't a legitimate reason to turn down food, especially when a food pusher was being insistent.

"What if you were a vegetarian," I asked, "and Suzanne was pushing those trendy cookies with bacon in them. Would you eat them anyway?"

"Oh, no," she responded. "I wouldn't."

"Why?"

"Because I just wouldn't. If I were vegetarian, I wouldn't *consider* eating meat."

"And what if you had a peanut allergy, and there could be serious consequences if you ate anything with nuts in it? Would you give in if she made baked goods made with nuts, and then pushed and pushed you to have some?"

"Definitely not. It wouldn't matter how much she pushed. I would definitely say no."

"So you'd feel it was legitimate to say no to Suzanne if you were a vegetarian or if you had a peanut allergy?"

"I would."

"Okay," I continued. "Let's talk about whether your goal of losing weight is also legitimate." I asked Theresa to read her advantages list aloud. Along with many other positive consequences of losing weight, she had identified important ways her health stood to improve. "But even if you didn't get *any* health benefits as a result of losing weight, wouldn't it be legitimate for you to turn down food so you could feel better about yourself, have more self-confidence, and feel strong and in control?"

She nodded. "Yes, I guess I hadn't been thinking about it that way."

"And what if the shoe were on the other foot? What if Suzanne had a goal to lose weight so she could get these advantages? Would you push food on her?"

"No," Theresa answered. "I'd respect her decision."

Theresa summarized her thoughts on a reminder card:

It's legitimate for me to say no! I'm fully within my rights to turn down food so I can lose weight and get the benefits of weight loss—just like I'd be fully within my rights to turn down food if I were vegetarian or had a food allergy. If Suzanne and I switched roles, I certainly wouldn't push food on her. I shouldn't let her push food on me.

Escape the Illegitimate to Say No Trap

Sometimes we have trouble seeing our own goals as worthy of as much respect as other people's preferences. And we don't realize that most people don't let others push them around when it comes to food. A lot of people are naturally good at standing firm if eating certain foods goes against their religious or philosophical practices or health needs. Others have no trouble putting their foot down if they're trying to lose or maintain their weight, or if they simply don't want the food.

- Consider the legitimacy of your weight-loss goal. You're entitled to resist food pushers and gain the benefits on your advantages list.

- Recognize that you have been acting as if the food pusher's (often thoughtless) desires are more legitimate than your goals for yourself.

- Think of determined food pushers as bullies. Would you bully someone else about food?

- Consider who might be a good role model for you in a food-pushing situation. Ask yourself, "If [Uncle Jim] were offered food he didn't want, what would he do? And if a food pusher really pushed? What would he say to stand firm?"

#6: The Willing Accomplice Trap

You don't put up much of a fight because, truthfully, you want to eat!

Some dieters don't protest food pushers' behavior because they actually *want* the food or drink that's being pushed on them. I asked Theresa if she ever fell in that category, too.

Theresa thought about it. "Yes," she said. "Sometimes. I really get tempted by her desserts."

"So what do you think?" I asked. "You could plan in advance to have the dessert she's offering instead of eating your own dessert after dinner. That way you'd be eating what you're supposed to eat."

Theresa considered this option. "I'm not sure. I really like saving dessert until after dinner. It helps to have a treat to look forward to all day. And it's not as if I never get to have Suzanne's desserts. We have dinner with my husband's family pretty often, and she always bakes then, too."

Theresa had to fortify her resolve in preparation for Suzanne's food pushing, especially when it came to desserts she really liked and wanted. She needed to practice a compelling response to her sabotaging thoughts. Being firm with a food pusher is much, much more difficult if you aren't firm with yourself first.

I suggested that Theresa ask herself, given all the variables involved, whether it was *worth it* to her to skip dessert after lunch at Suzanne's. She decided it was and made a reminder card:

> I can take control of the situation at Suzanne's. I've given in before, not only because she pushed me to eat her desserts but also because I really wanted to eat them. But even more, I want to be able to stay on track and lose weight. It's important to save my treat until after dinner, which is when I'll really enjoy it. Giving in once sets up a cycle of more giving in, which makes me feel terrible. It's worth it to resist!

Escape the Willing Accomplice Trap

As with all food pusher traps, you can be your own best advocate or you can be a pushover. But first you need to be clear about your own intentions. Are you giving in partly because you actually *want* to eat the food that's being pushed? Shortly before entering a situation with a known food pusher:

- Develop a strong plan for what you will and won't eat. Write it down and carry it with you. Spend a few moments seriously reflecting on your full advantages list. Make sure it's crystal clear why it's *worth it* to you to turn down food the food pusher is insisting you eat, especially if the food is enticing.

- Review relevant reminder cards. (If you're feeling especially vulnerable, put them in your pocket or purse, and steal into the bathroom for a quick booster during the meal.)

- Remember, you won't be firm with someone else if you're not first firm with yourself. Be sure to give yourself *extra* credit when you do stand firm, with both yourself and the food pusher, and record that experience in your memory journal.

Creating Escape Plans for Food Pushers

Most everyone has a food pusher in his or her life—but whether you get caught in a trap is entirely up to you. An escape plan can remind you that it is you—not anyone else—who is in charge of what goes into your body and can help you when you find your resolve weakening. As you become consistently assertive about your desires, you will find that other people are less likely to pressure you. You can start by creating your own escape plans:

❶ Identify a future situation in which a food pusher trap might arise.

❷ Record your sabotaging thoughts.

❸ Write a compelling response to each sabotaging thought.

❹ Develop a list of strategies.

❺ Review and revise your escape plan often.

Consider the following sample escape plan as you brainstorm and craft your own.

Escape Plan: Food Pusher Trap

Situation #1: GNO—Girls' Night Out with Jackie. I love her, but it's hard to stick to my plan when we're out together.

Sabotaging Thoughts	Reminders	Strategies
Jackie will be too insistent. If I order a burger or cheese steak, she won't tease me about my diet. I can't let her drink alone—she'd think I was judging her. I feel like I'm being such a downer when I order a salad on GNO—these nights are for indulgence! Splitting 2 desserts is "our thing," and I don't want to spoil it.	I can be just as insistent back. I don't want to be sorry later for giving in. Eating to avoid teasing is a habit I need to break. Jackie is a good friend. I can talk to her in advance about what I'm planning to do. It's not all or nothing. I can plan to have one drink. Besides, she knows me well enough to know that I do my best not to judge people, least of all her. If I want to lose weight, I can't eat the way I used to. The indulgence is being out together without kids and without husbands! It's not like I'd spoil the whole GNO. We can still split one dessert. If she's disappointed, she'll get over it. Don't use Jackie as an excuse if I secretly want to overindulge anyway.	Stand up to Jackie. Tell her before we go that I'm only going to have one drink and split one dessert. If she protests, tell her I want to focus on having fun with her, not on the food. Order one drink, then club soda. Or 2 wine spritzers. Decide in advance whether to order an entrée salad and eat most of it or something more caloric and eat less of it. Give myself credit for changing GNO in a way that will make me proud of myself when I leave the restaurant instead of regretful.

Reflect and Recommit:
Why I Want to Escape This Trap

Food pushers are just people; they are not superior beings, and you don't have to let them control what you put in your mouth. If you keep giving in to food pushers, you'll continue to suffer the consequences. Or you can decide to make a change.

What has happened in the past in your interactions with food pushers? What's likely to happen now and in the future if you don't become more assertive? **If you just say no (repeatedly if needed), will the world come to an end?**

Think about your next meeting with a known food pusher. How can you prepare yourself? Take a few minutes to write one final summary reminder card to motivate you to make changes and keep making changes.

Chapter 6

Family Traps

Eating with your family—whether it's the one you grew up with, your extended family, or your partner or kids—can be fraught with difficulty. Interacting with family members around food can lead to a variety of traps for dieters who are valiantly trying to stick to their plan.

If you have an "everyone-gets-along" family, eating occasions can be pleasant and fun, and you may not have too much difficulty sticking to your eating plan. Unless . . .

Unless there are loads of enticing treats that you crave.

Unless you're tempted to eat like family members who *aren't* actively trying to watch their weight.

Unless you're tempted to keep drinking or eating to keep a good time going.

Another problem may arise at home, even if your partner or family is relatively supportive. You may have trouble convincing yourself that you are *entitled* to make necessary changes, either temporary or long-term ones, especially if the changes affect the rest of the family. For example, many dieters change when they eat, what they eat, and the food they keep in the house. Or they may change who is responsible for shopping, preparing, or cleaning up after meals. But to make these changes, they have to feel entitled to do so.

When family members are difficult, the problems become even more challenging. Maybe certain people in your family don't want you to make changes, even when they recognize that those changes could help you. Spouses or partners can grow attached to "the way things are." Or maybe they fear you'll lose weight and then lose interest in them. Children are not known for happily relinquishing junk food or unlimited access to certain foods. Your parents and grandparents may toss around a bit of guilt if you try to make changes in family eating rituals. Siblings and cousins may not want to face the uncomfortable realization that they should really change their eating, too. You may encounter all kinds of resistance or be subject to unkind, demoralizing remarks: "Why even bother? You know you're never going to lose weight. You always gain it back."

To overcome complex, recurring family traps, you need to have a plan that will help you respond to your sabotaging thoughts while you also become more assertive with your loved ones. You can fine-tune strategies by learning about the most common family traps.

#1: The Criticizer Trap

You have unsupportive family members who make negative comments.

Growing up in a small town in Connecticut, Mia always dreamed of the day she would be able to move out of her parents' house. As a teenager, she had had a stormy relationship with both her mother and father, and she couldn't wait to go away to college. Once she did, she never lived at home again, but she still visited occasionally—and every visit was a fresh reminder of why Mia had been so desperate to leave.

As a lawyer living in Manhattan, Mia loved the energy and vibrancy of her chosen city but found it difficult to balance healthy eating and exercise with a demanding job. She loved to eat, and her weight had always been an issue growing up. Some of her oldest, clearest memories were of being told by her mother on a daily basis that she was too heavy. Her mother constantly directed Mia's eating: when she should eat, what she should eat, and how much she should eat. She let Mia's sister, who didn't have a weight problem, have dessert, but not Mia—which made Mia angry. At our first session (held via Skype), Mia told me she was more than eighty pounds overweight.

When we first started working with dieters, we were struck by how thoughtless, critical, or downright mean family members can be about body weight and appearance. We recognized that we could talk endlessly about how our clients' upbringing contributed to their current weight problems—but such a focus would do little to help them lose weight *now*. Instead we found that the most effective approach was to focus on how to respond to the cutting remarks that dieters still hear, to learn how to let those remarks roll off their backs, and to stick to their plans anyway.

Mia had clearly been hurt by her mother's comments over the years, but she began to understand that she couldn't change the past, only the present. She agreed to work on learning how to handle her mother now.

After four months of working together, Mia had lost nearly fifteen pounds. Now she was worried about how to handle a visit home to celebrate her father's birthday. "I'm sure Mom will say things like, 'Your clothes are looking too tight' or 'You're not really going to have a second helping, are you?' The last time I was home, she came down to the kitchen around ten at night and saw me taking a brownie, and she said, 'I think you're just fooling yourself if you think you'll ever lose weight eating like that.'"

"Being at home sounds like it must be *really* difficult," I sympathized. "Can we start with how to handle your mom's comments?" When Mia agreed, I asked her what she'd *like* to be able to say.

"Well, I'd like to say that she needs to mind her own business!"

I nodded. "I'm not surprised you would! How do you think she'd react if you said that?"

"Not well," she sighed. "She'd probably get defensive and go around in a huff the whole rest of the time I'm there." After thinking for a few moments, Mia said, "I guess it would be better to say, 'Please don't make any comments about my weight. When you say something about my eating, it's just counterproductive.'"

Mia decided she would try to forestall her mother's negative comments by saying that exact sentence to her over the phone before she left New York. "And if she starts in with me, I'll tell her to stop." She smiled. "As a lawyer, I've learned how to be firm." To help her prepare for the visit, Mia made the following list:

Weekend Visit Home

1. Call Mom before the weekend. Tell her I know she's concerned about my weight—but it's just counterproductive when she says anything about my eating.

2. If she protests, nicely but firmly say, "Please stop. I don't want to discuss it."

3. Then change the subject—ask her about the weekend plans or how other family members are doing.

Then we discussed what Mia could do if she was still bothered by her mother's comments even after they had changed the subject. Mia realized that she would need to get her mind off what her mother had said. I told her that some people find it helpful to imagine that comments like these are just insignificant little raindrops sliding down a windshield or off a raincoat into oblivion. Mia liked this metaphor and created a visual image of raindrops sliding down her shiny new white raincoat and falling right off. She added this item to her list.

4. If Mom makes comments, take control of the situation. Refuse to talk about it and then let her comments roll off my back, like raindrops off my new raincoat.

A few days after our session, Mia told me that she had unexpectedly gotten a chance to practice her new strategy. Her mother had called, announced that she was coming to town, and told Mia she wanted to have dinner with her. Mia was pleased with how she handled herself at the restaurant. She was able to limit her mother's negative remarks by being assertive and changing the subject. And then she was able to put on her "raincoat" and let her mother's comments roll off her back. She really took control of the situation.

Escape the Criticizer Trap

The criticizer can vary from well meaning but misguided to downright cruel, with many shades in between. Start with these suggestions.

Whether or not you can stop offensive comments, you can certainly change your reaction to them.

- Directly ask your family members not to make comments. For example, if they're skeptical about whether you'll succeed this time, you could say, "Time will tell, but in the meantime, please don't make any more comments about this."

- Create a visual image so you can "put on your raincoat" or "turn on the windshield wipers" and have critical comments harmlessly slide away.

- When family members say things that undermine your confidence in being able to lose weight, remind yourself, "This time is different—I'm learning skills I never had before."

- If the family members making unhelpful comments are not mean spirited, remind yourself that they may actually believe they *are* being helpful. They may not be intentionally trying to anger or demoralize you. But that doesn't necessarily mean you should accept their unhelpful remarks without saying anything.

- Remember, you are in charge of your reaction. You can choose to let what others say throw you off track and interfere with your goal of losing weight—*or* you can decide not to let the comments get in the way and continue following your plan.

#2: The Rebel Trap

You revert to old behaviors when interacting with your family.

Many adults naturally revert to childlike behavior when they are with their family. If you spent your childhood and teen years being told what to eat and what not to eat or feeling criticized about your appearance, you may find yourself rebelling many years later when you're around your family. This trap occurs when the rebellious choices you make sabotage your efforts. Ironically, if you have a knee-jerk reaction to your family and engage in unhealthy eating that drives you farther from your goals, you're not making free, independent choices. You're still being controlled.

The potential for rebellion was another problematic aspect of Mia's trip. "Historically, even when my eating has been more or less okay in my everyday life, I tend to lose control when I go home," she said. "I just regress back to old bad habits." When she was a teen, Mia hid food in her room or secretly slipped downstairs after everyone had gone to bed to eat chocolate chips or other junk food from the pantry. Every day she'd spend her lunch money on french fries and a milk shake. Even now, fifteen years later, those habits often came back when she returned home. On the drive to her parents' house, she would stop to buy treats to hide in her room, and sometimes she would sneak downstairs at night to eat leftovers from the fridge and food from the pantry. She felt a strong urge to rebel whenever she saw her mother watching what she ate.

Mia needed to keep in mind that though she was not able to make all her own eating decisions when she was a kid, she was absolutely in control now. Her mother no longer had the power to dictate what she did and didn't eat. She created the following reminder card:

I am an adult and I make all my own food decisions. Mom no longer has the power to make them for me, so there's nothing to rebel against anymore. If I have a knee-jerk reaction to her and rebel by overeating, it only hurts me. It's _my_ goal to lose weight.

Mia told me that even though she knew she shouldn't, she was still tempted to bring junk food with her. Her sabotaging thought was "If I have a rotten time at home, at least I'll have some treats to eat at night and feel better." But Mia recognized that she would only feel better for the few minutes the food was in her mouth. She knew she'd feel guilty and bad afterward. On the other hand, if she stayed in control at night, she'd feel better about herself, which would give her extra strength to deal with her parents. To help her remember this positively reinforcing cycle, Mia made the following reminder card:

> Eating junk food at night while I'm at home only makes me feel worse, not better. Staying in control of my eating will make me feel great and strong and make it easier for me to deal with everything else. Going home is hard enough. Don't make it even harder by getting off track with my eating.

Part of Mia's night eating was also a classic "fooling yourself" sabotaging thought: "It's okay to eat [this junk food] because no one is watching." Rationally, Mia knew that didn't make sense, but she found that particular sabotaging thought hard to shake. What helped Mia with this thought was reminding herself that calories are calories. It didn't matter whether her mom knew about the secret eating or not. If she ate too much, she'd gain weight. Period. She captured this important idea on another reminder card:

> If I eat extra, unplanned calories in secret at night, I _will_ gain weight, whether or not Mom knows about it. My body processes all calories the same whether 100 people are watching me eat or no one is watching me eat.

Once we had the major hurdles worked out, Mia and I discussed a few additional strategies for her list. She wouldn't be able to leave work until after seven o'clock on Friday. She knew she'd be hungry on the road and would be tempted to stop for junk food. To avoid this temptation, Mia decided she would bring a healthy and satisfying snack from home to eat right before she got on the road.

Mia had also been walking every day before work. She knew it would feel good to get in some exercise during the weekend. We decided that it would be important for her to get out of the house and take at least one walk on Saturday and again on Sunday, for three reasons: as a stress reliever and a chance to regroup; to maintain her exercise habit, regardless of the circumstances; and to prove to herself that she *could* change old patterns from her childhood and institute new and healthy ones *that she herself chose*. Finally, Mia and I discussed what she could do if she had nighttime cravings. She added these items to her list.

Weekend Visit Home

1. Bring a healthy snack from home to eat before I get on the road.

2. Don't stop and buy junk food; eating it will just make me feel worse.

3. If I'm tempted to sneak downstairs at night and eat, look at my old high school yearbooks or diaries. Choose one of my favorite childhood books to reread.

4. Go for at least one 30-minute walk a day.

5. Read this list and my advantages list and reminder cards at least 3 times a day, starting on Friday.

6. Make sure to give myself extra credit for every skill I practice and every good eating decision I make this weekend.

When Mia and I had another Skype session a few days later, she told me she was really proud of herself. Her experience going home had been more rewarding than usual. Though she still had some difficult nonfood interactions with her mom, she stayed in control of her eating.

The hardest part, she confessed, was when she was lying in her old bed on Saturday night, tempted by the leftover triple-chocolate birthday cake downstairs in the kitchen. "But I read my reminder cards and reminded myself that eating it would make me feel worse, not better. I picked up *Little Women* and got engrossed in it, and the urge to eat the cake went away. I was so glad that I didn't eat it!"

Mia said she felt much more comfortable and confident with her eating because she had a plan and knew she would be equipped to handle the difficult parts. She recorded how happy she felt in her memory journal and what she had done to make the weekend such a success. She carefully saved her list for her next trip home.

Escape the Rebel Trap

When it comes to rebellion, you can be your own worst enemy (you, and not anyone else, because you're in control of every bite of food you put in your mouth). When you tend toward self-sabotage, the best overall strategy is to continually question your unhelpful thinking and remind yourself, "If I do this, whom will my overeating actually affect? Won't I really just be hurting myself? What does my adult mind say about this?"

- Remember that you've grown up and you are now responsible for making your own food decisions. It's up to you whether you let difficult family interactions affect your eating.

- Keep in mind that it doesn't matter if you eat in secret or in front of other people. If you take in too many calories, you'll gain weight. Your body registers every bite.

- Read your reminder cards whenever you're tempted to rebel by eating.

- Give yourself credit for dealing with your rebellious self-sabotage.

- Note your successes over self-sabotage in your memory journal.

#3: The Can't Deprive the Family Trap

You keep tempting foods at home because you don't want your family to "suffer."

Maxine worked for a local nonprofit organization and was devoted to her three kids and their many activities. Preparing meals they really enjoyed and stocking the house with snacks they asked for were ways she communicated her love, just as her mother had done when Maxine was growing up. But it was also a way Maxine sabotaged the goal she had for herself to eat in a more healthy way and lose weight.

Potato chips were Maxine's nemesis. Maxine continued to buy a large bag of chips for the family during her major shopping trip of the week even though they were a constant temptation and often got the better of her. "It's ridiculous—I'm constantly finishing a bag, and then I have to buy another one so my family doesn't realize they're gone, and then I finish the new bag. And so I usually end up buying a third bag. It's really a problem."

I told Maxine that the buy-eat-buy cycle was not ridiculous when you considered that the potato chip industry expressly engineers chips to be as tempting as possible. I assured her that almost every successful dieter and maintainer has at least one extremely tempting food that they limit or keep out of the house entirely, either temporarily or permanently. "For me it used to be cashews," I told her. "It wasn't that I couldn't learn to eat cashews in reasonable portions, and ultimately I did. But at one point it was a struggle, so I just didn't buy them for a while. I figured, why make things harder than they need to be?"

Maxine recognized that keeping lots of potato chips around the house sabotaged her weight-loss efforts and she needed to stop, at least until her resistance muscle got stronger. But she struggled with the idea of telling her kids that she was planning a change. Lots of sabotaging thoughts got in the way:

"I don't want to deprive the kids."

"They won't like not having potato chips around."

"Why should they suffer because I can't control myself?"

We talked about the fact that this wasn't an all-or-nothing situation: it wasn't as if there had to be a big bag of potato chips in the house or none at all. But Maxine didn't think buying packs of single-serve bags of potato chips would work; she might be tempted to eat several bags at a time. We came up with a new idea. The kids could buy chips for lunch at school or just one single-serve bag at the convenience store to eat as a snack that day. When Maxine thought about it, she realized that they would probably even prefer to buy the kind of chips they wanted.

The more we talked, the more Maxine recognized that of course her kids wouldn't suffer if she stopped buying large bags of chips. She also wasn't depriving them of healthy food (quite the contrary, in fact). Maxine composed a reminder card so she wouldn't falter when broaching the change with her kids:

> *I need to tell the family that we won't be having big bags of potato chips in the house, at least for a while. The kids can buy chips themselves, and they'd probably prefer that anyway. They won't suffer. Not having a big bag of chips won't deprive them of any important nutrients.*

Escape the Can't Deprive the Family Trap

Even people with supreme self-discipline often have a weakness for certain foods. And no law dictates that you *have* to provide your family with any particular food. Your sabotaging thoughts can really interfere with making changes that are important if you are to reach your goal of long-lasting weight loss.

- Assess how big a sacrifice it will really be for your family if you keep difficult-to-resist foods out of the house, at least temporarily. Compare that with the potential benefit for you.

- If you decide to have these foods in your house, consider keeping only single-serving packages, if you can limit yourself to just one.

- Store these foods in places you can't see or easily access. Research has demonstrated that you are much more likely to achieve your goals if you avoid visual cues. And while out of sight is out of mind, out of the house is even better.

#4: The Me-First Mule Trap

Stubborn or controlling family members don't want to make changes.

In some cases, loved ones react poorly when you ask for changes. Perhaps your spouse or partner feels threatened by your weight loss; if you get too thin, you might leave him. Or maybe she sees your efforts to get healthy as an unwelcome mirror for her own unhealthy habits—and she'd rather sabotage you than make changes herself. If those scenarios sound accurate, you probably have a genuine me-first mule in your house, and you may need stronger strategies.

Me-first mules are on a continuum of difficulty. The easier ones are family members who are flexible in other areas but insist on their way when it comes to decisions about food. The ones who present the most difficulty are those who are controlling about many issues, including food—the "my-way-or-the-highway" type.

Characterized by stubbornness and immobility, me-first mules insist that their approach to food must reign supreme. They resist your requests to make changes. If you are not already assertive in other areas, you will need to learn this essential interpersonal skill to negotiate changes with the me-first mule.

It turned out that Maxine's biggest family trap was not her kids; it was her husband, Mike. Mike regularly arrived home from his second-shift job after their youngest child was in bed. As a result, Maxine ate dinner with her children at five-thirty and then ate more a few hours later with Mike. And because Claire, at age thirteen, had become even pickier about her eating, Maxine often ended up preparing two separate meals.

Maxine had been a little vague describing her food intake in the evenings, so I asked her to keep track of everything she ate from the time she got home from work until she went to bed. When she returned for the next session, she was aghast. "I considered dinner with the kids as my major meal. I thought I was just nibbling when I sat down with Mike at nine o'clock—but I guess I wasn't paying enough attention to how much I was eating." She found although she didn't eat as much as Mike did, she was having almost a second meal.

We started by discussing some solutions. Maxine could eat a full meal with the kids and just have a snack with her husband. She could eat a snack with her kids and dinner with her husband. Or she could have half a meal at each.

"If you knew your family wouldn't give you a hard time, which would you choose?" I asked.

Maxine thought about it. "Well, I'm really hungry when I get home from work and I'm ready for dinner, so I guess I wouldn't choose to have a snack or half a meal with the kids. But . . ." Maxine hesitated. When I asked her what was going through her mind, she expressed a sabotaging thought: "If I don't eat a whole meal with Mike, he won't be happy."

Maxine had evidence that this thought was true—Mike had expressed annoyance the few times she had told him she wasn't hungry at nine and didn't want to eat. "He doesn't want me to just sit there. He doesn't like to be the only one eating. When I brought it up with him, he said I shouldn't eat with the kids; I should wait for him."

"Does it have to be all or nothing?" I asked. "What would you think about having one food when you sit with him—maybe a salad or a piece of fruit?"

"Hmmm." She pondered this option and sighed again. "He still won't be happy about it. He's always saying that the food is so good and I have to try some of this or that."

"And how happy are you about the effects of eating with him so he'll be happy? How happy are you that it's difficult to carry laundry baskets up and down the basement stairs?"

She shook her head.

"How happy are you that the doctor has told you your blood pressure is too high? Or that you decided not to go to the pool last weekend because you don't have a bathing suit that fits?"

"Not happy at all," she admitted. "In fact, pretty unhappy, I guess."

"How come it's okay for you to feel unhappy—but not him?"

We sat in silence for a few moments while Maxine reflected on this question. "I see what you mean," she said finally. "I guess I do see that being healthier should be more important than making Mike happy by eating dinner with him."

Maxine created the following reminder card:

If Mike is disappointed that I'm not eating more, that's okay. My goal of being healthier is more important.

Then Maxine said, "Okay, I'll talk to him. But I'm not sure what I should say." I suggested we role-play. I would be Maxine, and Maxine would be Mike.

I started. "Mike, when we sit down in a few minutes, I'm just going to have a salad. That's going to be my plan because I can't be healthy if I eat with the kids and then eat again with you."

"But you know I like it when we eat together," Maxine said, crossing her arms. "Why don't you skip eating with the kids so you can eat with me?"

"Well, I'd be willing to try that once in a while," I said. "But it really works out better for me to eat at five-thirty when I'm hungry. I don't need all the extra food later on."

Maxine scowled. "But you know it's not much fun eating by myself."

"I know. That's why I'm going to save part of my meal to eat with you. I'm just not going to have another *full* meal."

Maxine pursed her lips, looking exasperated. "Can't you work it out another way?"

"It's possible, but this seems like my best bet to lose weight."

Her voice softened a bit. "Come on, you don't really have to lose weight."

"Yes, I do. It's not healthy for me to be at this weight. And I keep gaining every year. I know you don't like it when I don't go to the beach or when I get so out of breath I can't help you outside."

"I can rake and shovel by myself. You don't need to help."

"Thank you, but I don't want this to get any worse. I *really* want it to get better."

"Well, I don't know. I don't like the idea."

"I know. But I'd like to try it for two weeks and see how it goes. Okay, are you ready for dinner now?"

Role-playing helped Maxine feel more confident about standing up to Mike. She committed to her plan by making a list.

Eating Dinner with Mike

1. Tell Mike my plan will be to have a salad with him because

   - It's not healthy for me to continue to gain weight every year.
   - My blood pressure is too high and I get out of breath too easily.
   - It's getting hard to carry the laundry up and down the steps.

2. Tell him I want to try this for 2 weeks.

3. Then change the subject.

I sensed that Maxine needed more fortification. I asked her if she could think of a time when she stood up to her husband on a nonfood matter. She thought about it. "Yes, a couple of weeks ago. Mike wanted to take our son Tim to a movie that I thought would be too scary. Mike was pretty stubborn, but he did listen to reason."

"Great example," I said. "So if you feel like backing down about the two-dinner issue, can you remind yourself of how successful you were in standing up to Mike to protect Tim?" Maxine summarized our discussion on a reminder card:

I stood up to Mike for Tim's sake, and I can stand up to him on my own behalf. This shows me that when I think something is important, I can do it!

When Maxine returned the following week, I asked her how it had gone. "Actually, he seemed a little surprised that I stood up to him. He did give me kind of a hard time at first. But I stuck to my guns and limited myself to just a salad every night. And now I think he accepts it."

"That's terrific!" I replied. It was a real triumph for Maxine, the first of several. Mike gave her plenty of opportunities to practice being assertive. He was really a classic example of a me-first mule.

Escape the Me-First Mule Trap

If you have never lived with someone like Mike, you might think that Maxine is a pushover. But take a look at your interactions with family members; you may find some similarities. If you have a me-first mule in your life, you need to learn to be assertive. You may never be able to convince the mule to consider the needs of others in the stable. But if you are firm and persistent, you can nicely and assertively insist on making changes that are important for your well-being. Some of the following tips may apply in your situation:

- If you think it will help, talk about the importance of your being healthy and how being unhealthy is negatively affecting you in specific ways (and if relevant, how it's negatively affecting others, especially the me-first mule).

- If necessary, start with a compromise—getting part of the change you need—and then over time introduce additional changes. For example, you might start by telling your meat-and-potatoes spouse that you want to eat a little lighter once a week. Then you could move up to two or three times a week. Small steps may be the way to go with me-first mules who are adamantly against changes they don't initiate, especially wholesale changes.

- Practice your skills with a friend by role-playing a potential confrontation with your me-first mule. Ask your friend to act stubborn so you can practice being persistent. (If you get stuck, reverse roles and ask her what she would say.) Write down important points.

- Visualize yourself being assertive and rehearse assertive statements to gain the strength and stamina not to back down. Assertiveness is not an inborn trait; it's a learned skill.

- Consider telling the me-first mule that you will make the change for a short time (perhaps two weeks or a month) and then reevaluate.

#5: The Me-Last Martyr Trap

You feel unentitled to ask family members to make changes.

Some people tend to get stuck in a "you first / me last" pattern. Constantly putting others first can become such an ingrained habit that you don't even recognize that you've been relegating your own needs to the bottom of the list.

When Maxine and I began to discuss her difficulties, it became apparent that she was still a me-last martyr. She knew intellectually that it was problematic for her, for example, to cook a different meal for her daughter, Claire, or to go out for ice cream with Mike and the kids on Saturday afternoons. But she still believed that she should make everyone happy.

"Could these problems be new examples of how you put everyone else's *desires* ahead of your *needs*?" I asked. "Claire doesn't *need* you to cook her a separate meal. Mike doesn't *need* you to get ice cream with him and the kids. But *you need* to eat differently to keep healthy." I let her think about this for a moment. "Protecting your health isn't just a desire to eat differently," I continued. "It's a need. What do you think will happen if you don't start putting your needs above some of their desires? Aren't you entitled to ask your family to make changes?"

Maxine sighed. Standing up for herself was still difficult. But she could see that it would be necessary if she were to lose weight. "I guess it's okay to do what I need to do—even if they don't like it. The kids did get used to the potato chip rule. Mike doesn't complain much anymore about my eating only a salad with him."

"Exactly!" I said. "And it's not just okay but important!" I reminded Maxine that she wasn't asking her family to make changes to make them unhappy; she was asking them to make changes so she could reach extraordinarily important goals, so she could safeguard her health.

> My _needs_ are more important than my family's wants. I'm entitled to institute changes so I can reach important goals. Not making changes hasn't worked. Even if they don't like the changes, they'll eventually get used to them.

Over the next few weeks, Maxine gradually introduced additional changes—some temporary and others permanent. For example, she decided to cook just one meal for everyone. She got Claire to help her make dishes that they could freeze in single portions (lasagna, for example) for Claire to heat in the microwave for herself. And Claire always had the option of making herself a sandwich.

As time went on, Maxine slowly began to identify her needs and implement the necessary changes. Putting herself first became easier, especially when she realized that her family adapted to a new status quo fairly quickly.

Escape the Me-Last Martyr Trap

Do you fall into this trap? Sometimes putting yourself last is so habitual that you don't even realize you're doing it. To identify the changes you need to make, imagine an alternate reality. If you knew for sure that your family would happily go along with anything you wanted, what would you do differently?

- Consider how the status quo has been interfering with your ability to lose weight.

- Identify sabotaging thoughts. Do you believe, for example, that you have to make your family happy no matter what? If you're hesitant to put yourself first, ask yourself, "Isn't it okay for family members to be inconvenienced or slightly uncomfortable for an important cause?"

- Assess whether you're viewing changes in an all-or-nothing way. Are you assuming that any change you make has to be permanent or not at all? Or that if they're not happy about a change now, they'll never accept it?

Creating Escape Plans for Family Traps

Maxine's and Mia's stories are classic family dilemmas we see quite often in our practice. History, personalities, and family dynamics can make family interactions and gatherings into a minefield when you're trying to lose weight. Still, the foundation strategies and the strategies in this chapter can help you solve family problems, whether they're related to others' comments and actions or to your own sabotaging thoughts and behavior.

Create your own escape plans:

❶ Identify a future situation in which a family trap might arise.

❷ Record your sabotaging thoughts.

❸ Write a compelling response to each sabotaging thought.

❹ Develop a list of strategies.

❺ Review and revise your escape plan often.

Consider the following sample escape plan as you brainstorm and craft your own.

Escape Plan: Family Trap

Situation #1: Baking cookies with Mom. I will be tempted to eat too much. She will insist that I take lots of cookies home with me and may criticize me if I don't.

Sabotaging Thoughts	Reminders	Strategies
I love cookie dough. I hardly ever get the chance to have it. It won't matter if I have it. And Mom is having some, too. I'll hurt Mom's feelings if I tell her I'm not taking any cookies home. Mom will be so disappointed if I don't take cookies home. I shouldn't disappoint her. Mom will criticize me if I tell her I'm not taking cookies home or if I tell her I'm trying to lose weight.	Since my goal is to lose weight, IT DOES MATTER if I eat too much cookie dough. Every time I get off track with my eating, I make it so much more likely that I'll get off track the next time, too. How much cookie dough Mom eats will have zero effect on the weight that I'll gain if I eat more than I planned. I'm an adult. I need to make decisions that are in line with goals that are important to me. It's okay if Mom is disappointed. Her disappointment will be minor and fleeting. If I eat too much, my disappointment will be huge. Mom may criticize me, but so what if she does. I can ask her to stop. Roy would have no problem saying that to her.	Eat a good lunch before I go and read my advantages list and reminder cards. Plan to have 1 tablespoon of cookie dough and 3 cookies, but eat them sitting down. Call Mom now and tell her I'd love to bake with her but I won't be taking any cookies home. Use Roy as my role model. If she criticizes me, be nice but firm, ask her to stop, then quickly change the subject. Set a new standard of not letting Mom push food on me. If I don't want to take any cookies home, that means I'm definitely not taking them home. Give myself lots of credit for sticking up for myself.

Reflect and Recommit:
Why I Want to Escape This Trap

You can keep denying your own needs to keep your family happy—but be ready to keep yourself unhappy in the process. You deserve to do what you need to do to lose weight and become healthier. You can learn to make changes that protect your needs, even in moments of conflict or power struggle.

What has happened in the past in your interactions with difficult family members? Have you given in? What's likely to happen in the future if you don't change? Why do you act as if it's more important to fulfill other people's desires instead of taking care of yourself? **Why do other people deserve your care, but not you?**

Take a long, hard look at some of the family traps you've encountered, so you can have a head start on the next family conflict. Take a few minutes to write one final summary reminder card to help motivate you to make changes and keep making changes.

PART FOUR

External Traps: How Special Circumstances Trap Me

Chapter 7

Travel and Eating Out Traps

E ating away from home can be one of life's pleasures, but it presents lots of opportunities for falling into a trap, especially if you tell yourself:

"It's a special meal. I can loosen up."

"I deserve to eat what I want."

"Eating out should be different from eating in."

"It's my vacation! I shouldn't have to limit myself."

Eating out can be challenging for many reasons, whether you're close to home, dining at restaurants or at the homes of family or friends, or traveling for vacation or business. You may have more choices of what to eat and drink and be sorely tempted by the sheer variety of what is available. You might be dining at different hours, with different people, and in new restaurants and settings, all of which can stimulate you to make exceptions that you'll be sorry for later. At the same time, you usually don't have control over how the food is prepared or the size of the portions you're served.

Dining at restaurants, with all their options, can be a wonderful experience but can also provide countless enticements. Perhaps you feel deprived if you don't have a "full" meal of wine, appetizer, bread, salad, entrée, *and* dessert. Maybe you think, "I have to get my money's worth" or "I can't leave food on my plate." Or you might say to yourself, "It's okay to eat like this today—I'll make up for it tomorrow."

To escape from these traps, you must learn how to make changes to your mind-set and plan ahead. Otherwise, you risk getting off track. You're likely to find yourself eating impulsively, enticed by the sight, smell, or menu description of tantalizing food, baskets of bread, and tempting, oversize portions. Let's take a closer look at a few of these hard-to-resist traps.

#1: The 24/7 Treat Trap

You think every meal out should be "special"— even when you eat out all the time.

A mom of two boys, Kate worked from home part time as a freelance writer. When she first came to see me, she was upset that in the past few months she had added many more pounds to her already overweight frame.

"Our house is being remodeled, and our contractor said it would take about three weeks to finish," she said. "But it's already been a month and they're not done. The kitchen is completely out of commission." As a result, they'd been eating out frequently.

She and her husband loved trying new restaurants both alone and with their boys. "It's getting pretty ridiculous, though," she said. "We're eating out nearly every night, and I always eat too much. I keep trying to get myself to order food that's healthier and lower in calories—but then I just don't follow through. Or if I do, I eat everything on my plate plus bread and dessert. It's just too much."

I asked her what thoughts went through her mind the last time she was at a restaurant and ordered something she later regretted. "Well," she replied, "something like 'I know I should get a salad, but I'm really hungry.'"

"When was the last time you left a restaurant feeling hungry?" I asked.

She thought for a moment. "That's a good question. I don't leave hungry—even when I have a salad, because I order one with protein.

Plus I always have a piece of bread or roll with butter, too." She stopped to think. "You know, I really do like salads, and I guess they do always fill me up. They just don't seem as appealing when I'm looking at all the other choices."

I asked her another question. "Has there ever been a time when you ordered a salad and once the meal was over, you thought to yourself, 'I regret eating that. I wish I had something more fattening'?"

"No, definitely not," she said. "I always feel good after eating something healthy."

Kate decided that she would make it a firm policy to look at the online menu ahead of time and decide *in advance* what she was going to order. She could order anything she wanted, though she would have to restrict portion sizes for dishes that were higher in calories.

I could tell she was really thinking. "I have a feeling I'll still struggle when I hear about the daily specials," she said, her forehead furrowed. "That's usually the exact moment when I tell myself, 'That sounds much better.' What I had planned to eat just doesn't seem as special."

I could absolutely see how that thought might undermine her resolve. But I knew that with the number of times they were eating out right now, she couldn't order something "special" each time, eat the whole meal, and still lose weight—or even maintain her weight. "You could give yourself a choice," I said. "You could decide at the last minute to have one of the special dishes or go with your original choice. But if you order a higher-calorie special, you won't be able to eat as much of it as you'd like. I wonder if it might be better, just for now, to avoid ordering the specials. Once you've gotten really good at other restaurant skills, we can work on spontaneous ordering." Kate agreed.

To help her recognize that eating out could still be special, we identified other aspects of the experience that were different and enjoyable, aside from the food:

- Spending time with family
- Having someone else do the cooking and serving
- Not having to do dishes
- Going to a new place to eat
- Getting to admire the decor
- People-watching

"You're right," Kate said. "The food isn't the only special part." Kate made the following reminder cards:

When I eat out, decide in advance what to order—and stick to it. Even if I think I'm really hungry and won't be satisfied, that's not true. I'm always satisfied!

The food is just one aspect of eating out. Even if what I get doesn't feel as exciting as the specials, it's still good food that I like. And every other part of eating out is still special (spending time with Matthew and the kids, not having to cook or serve or clean up, the decor, people-watching).

Escape the 24/7 Treat Trap

When eating out, keep in mind that you will be able to eat only slightly more than usual if your goal is to lose weight. Most restaurant meals have hidden calories. A dieter who owned a restaurant once told us some of their tricks; you wouldn't guess how much oil or butter is added to dishes to make them more delectable!

- If you can, look at the menu before you go and decide what to have. Put your plan in writing. Making a healthy decision when you are at your computer is much easier than when you are in the restaurant and influenced by what you see and smell. Once you get to the restaurant, you won't even have to look at the menu and be tempted by other options.

- If you don't have access to the menu, develop a general plan that's well balanced and not overly caloric.

- Be the first one to place your order, so you won't be influenced when you hear what others are having. If you're tempted to change your decision, ask yourself, "When the meal is over, do I want to feel full and good, or do I want to feel full (maybe overly full) and guilty?"

- Make reminder cards for any thoughts that might get in the way of your being able to stick to your plan. Read them, and your advantages list, before you go. If you're tempted to eat extra unplanned food, excuse yourself from the table and find a place to read them again.

- If you'll be tempted to eat larger portions than you planned, ask whether there are half portions. If not, ask the waiter to wrap up half the usual portion and serve you the other half. Or when your food is brought to the table, immediately move the extra portion you hadn't planned to eat to your bread plate or the side of your dinner plate.

- Consider ordering two healthy appetizers and a side salad instead of a main course. Then you won't be tempted by oversize portions.

- Remember that even if the food doesn't feel particularly special, other aspects of eating out can be special. Won't you enjoy the fact that someone else is cooking, serving, and cleaning up? How about the surroundings, the music, and the people-watching opportunity?

#2: The Cleanup Crew Trap

You eat food from other people's plates.

When Kate returned two weeks later, she told me she was doing much better with eating out, but one food continued to trip her up. "It seems like every single kid's meal comes with fries. I love fries, so every time I see them, I want them. It's a huge struggle." Kate needed a french fries plan.

We discussed the situation at length and realized that deciding in advance to just take a few fries from her kids' plates wouldn't work because she always ended up taking more (while still eating everything else she had planned). Kate settled on the first part of her plan: "No fries from my kids' plates." Cut and dried. Very simple.

Kate and I agreed that it was reasonable for her to eat fries some of the time—just not *all* the time. She decided that she would plan *in advance* whether she was going to have fries at the meal. If her meal didn't come with them, she would order her *own* side dish of fries, even though her kids were unlikely to finish all of theirs.

Getting her own portion reinforced the message that she never ate fries from her kids' plates. Kate would have them only if she had decided in advance to get her own. She would also have to figure out how much of the portion to eat and adjust the rest of her meal accordingly. That way she wouldn't have to spend every meal deciding whether to grab some off the kids' plates—she would know she was not having any of theirs, period. No more struggle.

Kate and I then discussed what she could tell herself if she hadn't planned to order fries but wanted some. "I'll remind myself that fries will always be there! I don't have to have them every time. I know what they taste like, and I'll have them again."

Kate made the following reminder card:

> No matter what, no fries from the boys' plates. If I give in, it will be harder to stand firm the next time. I'm tired of the struggle, so I just have to give it up. Next time I can plan to get my own fries, but I'm not having theirs.

Kate then made a list.

The French Fries Plan

1. No fries from the boys' plates.

2. Decide in advance whether I'm going to order fries at that meal.

3. If I do, skip the other carbs.

4. If the portion of fries is too big, move the extra onto a different plate and push it away from me. Shake lots of pepper on the extra if I think I'll still be tempted.

5. Read my french fries reminder card before going out to eat.

With these strategies in place, Kate was finally able to follow her plan, and it made a big difference in both her weight and her confidence. She was no longer stressed or worried about how she would handle restaurant meals; she loved knowing that she could eat out and stay in control. "I still look at the boys' french fries and think they look good, but I just know I'm not having any of theirs. I've stopped struggling. It's really a great relief!"

Escape the Cleanup Crew Trap

When you eat out, going off plan is easy. You can be tempted by the menu, the looks and smells, the large portions, the food on everyone else's plates. If you're not fully committed to following your plan, you may either give up or feel constant tension. You may struggle with that uncomfortable "Should I? No, I shouldn't. But I really want to." And you run the risk of giving in.

Giving in leads to negative consequences, which you are probably trying not to think about at the moment of temptation. But the consequences are very real. You will make it harder for yourself to stay in control the next time. You will consume extra calories, which will slow your weight loss or lead to a weight gain. You will put a damper on your after-the-restaurant experience. How *do* you want to feel when you leave?

- Establish a firm guideline of not eating other people's food unless you've planned in advance to do so.

- Initiate a habit of ordering what you want for yourself, so you can end the struggle of "That looks so good. I really want it," and replace it with "I'm only eating what I ordered."

- If what you order is highly caloric or you're served too large a portion, plan to eat just part of it.

- If you're tempted by your dining companions' food, remind yourself that it is unlikely this will be the only opportunity in your life to have this food. You'll undoubtedly have a chance to have it again.

#3: Limited Food Options Trap

You don't have control over your food while on a trip.

Joe, a marketing executive, travels often for work, flying all around the country. As a result of frequent business dinners, unhealthy room service, and junky airport food, he has gained over forty pounds in the past ten years. When Joe first came to see me, he told me he was fed up with his increasing waistline but felt helpless to stop it. His wife was a healthy eater and cook, so eating at home wasn't usually a problem for him. Traveling was when he seemed to lose control.

"The problem starts right at the airport," he told me. "I'm always rushing, and I don't have time to look for healthy food, so I just grab fast food. It goes downhill from there."

I mentioned to Joe that I had seen a real change in airport food in the past few years. Now there are usually lots of healthy options. I suggested that if he couldn't get to the airport earlier next time, he could always get a prepackaged sandwich and a piece of fruit. When Joe agreed, I asked him to write a reminder card for his next trip:

Since I want to lose weight, I need to get a healthy sandwich at the airport. It doesn't take any more time. Fast food always makes me feel guilty and greasy, and it will make the time sitting on the airplane that much more unpleasant.

Joe told me about an upcoming business trip. "It's a large market-ing conference," he said. "We'll be meeting with lots of people in the industry and potential clients. I'll have business dinners to go to all four nights. And they put out all these sweet things for snacks, like doughnuts and pastries and muffins. I usually end up eating them, even though I know I shouldn't. But it's hard to get healthy snacks at these conferences."

We came up with a plan. If Joe was staying at a hotel with a gift shop, he could most likely buy nuts or protein bars—or just bring them from home. He pulled out his smartphone to add these items to his packing list. Noting that he's always busy just before traveling, he added a task into his schedule for the day before: "Buy nuts/bars."

Now we had to prepare Joe for sabotaging thoughts he might have when he saw people eating the conference snacks. "What do you want to remind yourself if you have your healthy snack with you but you're tempted by the doughnuts?" I asked.

Joe paused and thought. "I've had plenty of trips where I ate those snacks. They tasted good, but I felt bad afterward. And I gained weight. It really wasn't worth it." He wrote a reminder card:

No eating conference snacks! I don't want to feel bad, and I don't want to gain weight. Eating the healthy snacks I brought with me will make me feel good, and I won't gain weight. Win-win.

Joe's next problem would be conference dinners. "There's a set menu," he told me, "and you don't get much choice over what you eat."

I pointed out a very important distinction to Joe: while he may not always have control over what food is served to him, he *always* has the ability to control what food he actually puts in his mouth. Joe and I decided that during these conference dinners, he would make the best choices he could and institute portion control. Joe made a list.

Conference Dinner Plan

1. Club soda during cocktail hour

2. Up to 2 passed appetizers, plus raw vegetables if available

3. No bread (I have plenty of opportunities to get really good bread at home)

4. One glass of wine or beer during dinner

5. Salad with dressing on the side

6. Soup (but just a couple of spoonfuls if it's cream based)

7. Entrée (part of a portion if it's big) plus most of 2 side dishes

8. Reasonable-size portion of dessert, if it looks good

To help him stick to this plan, Joe made the following reminder card:

> *Remember, even though I don't always have control over what food is served to me, I always have control over what I put in my mouth. Stick to the plan and I'll feel good.*

One last aspect of business travel we needed to talk about involved the snacks the hotel provides in guest rooms. "I tend to eat them at night, even if I'm not really hungry, especially if I'm feeling keyed up or kind of bored. You know, they just sit there, on the minibar or counter, staring me in the face," he said.

Joe and I discussed potential solutions. He could ask the hotel to remove them. He could cover them with a towel. Or if they were on a tray, he could put them away in the closet.

"I like the idea of covering the snacks with a towel," Joe said to me. "Besides, I'm bringing healthy snacks with me, so I know I can eat those if I want to. And honestly, those minibar snacks are ridiculously expensive. Even though my business covers my expenses, I feel kind of ripped off."

To help him stick to this plan, Joe also made the following reminder card:

I'll be sorry if I eat the minibar snacks. If they weren't in the room at all, I wouldn't miss them.

To help him remember these strategies, Joe made the following list.

General Travel Plans

1. Bring healthy snacks.

2. If I have time to look for healthy food at the airport, that's fine. If not, grab a healthy sandwich or salad and fruit. I'll feel better if I do.

3. Limit food and drink at receptions and dinners. (See conference dinner plan.)

4. Cover the food on the hotel minibar. Out of sight, out of mind.

5. Read advantages list and reminder cards as usual every day.

6. Wake up early, if I need to, to exercise.

7. Walk whenever possible.

Escape the Limited Food Options Trap

Taking control of your eating on trips is a matter of preparation and practice. Think about all your meals and snacks. How can you get healthy food? How can you deal with temptations? Pull out your schedule, too. When can you fit in exercise?

- Save enough time so you can get something healthy to eat on the way to your destination. Remind yourself that it will probably take just as long to get a healthy option as it would to get junky food. Which will you feel better about having eaten?

- Bring healthy snacks with you or buy them at the hotel gift shop. Or when you check in, ask for directions to a food market and request a small refrigerator for your room. Ask the hotel to take away the mini-bar food or make sure it's out of sight.

- Before each meal, remind yourself that you don't always have control over what food is served to you, but you always have control over what food you put in your mouth.

- Make a specific plan for what to eat if you have an idea of what will be served. Make at least a general plan if you don't. How many courses will you eat? What will your portion sizes be?

- Schedule in times to exercise. Take advantage of exercise apps or on-demand exercise videos or explore the neighborhood—with the added benefit of getting some fresh air.

#4: The Vegas Mind-Set Trap

"What I eat on vacation stays on vacation."

Karen was excited. She was about to go to the beach for a week with her husband and three granddaughters. They had rented the same house at the Jersey shore each year for many years. Karen loved riding the waves with the kids, building sand castles, buying them treats from the bakery and the gift shops, eating out with the family, and visiting with neighbors and friends they had met through the years.

But Karen was worried. She had already lost thirty-five pounds and was concerned about what might happen next. On two-week beach vacations in the past, she had invariably gained about five pounds. And then when she got home, she struggled mightily to get back on track.

Karen's traditional mind-set had been, "I'm going on vacation. I deserve to loosen up. I don't want to ruin my trip by having to watch everything I eat." She told me it felt good to feel free to eat whatever she wanted. When I questioned her more closely, though, she realized that unrestrained eating didn't feel completely good. She actually felt guilty quite a lot. "And," she reflected, "when I have a big lunch, I feel heavier in my body. I feel pretty self-conscious when I change into a bathing suit and go to the beach."

I suggested that Karen write down the advantages and disadvantages of staying in control of her eating versus the advantages and disadvantages of following her customary habit of eating whatever she wanted. Here's what she came up with:

Advantages of eating whatever I want	Disadvantages of eating whatever I want
Feel freer	Always feel a little guilty
Don't have to think ahead and make a plan	Feel out of control
Can eat what everyone else is eating	Feel heavier in my body
Can eat more, especially my favorite foods that I don't usually let myself eat	Struggle with food decisions
	Feel more self-conscious in bathing suit
	Worry about whether I'll be able to get back in control when I get home
	Gain weight
	Undo my progress
	Reinforce bad eating habits
	Poor role model for kids
	Won't want family to know how much I'm eating so I'll sneak food, which feels bad
	Feel overstuffed at times, especially after big dinner and dessert

Advantages of staying in control	Disadvantages of staying in control
I'll feel better!	Can't eat spontaneously
Won't gain weight (or as much weight)	Have to plan in advance
Guilt won't interfere with the pleasure I do get from eating	Can't eat as much as I'd like
Will feel proud of myself	May have cravings
Won't have to worry about returning to everyday eating when I get home because I will have been on track the whole time	Won't be able to eat everything my family is eating
Won't dread getting on the scale when I get home	
Will feel lighter in my body	
Will feel less self-conscious	
Will be better role model for kids (not constantly snacking)	
Won't obsess about food and my weight, spoiling my fun	
Will feel more upbeat and positive during the trip because I won't be feeling bad about my eating	

When she finished the chart, Karen said, "Okay. It's clear. I guess it's exactly the same as at home. I feel better in control and worse when I'm out of control." She wrote herself a reminder card:

When I let my eating get out of control on vacation, it makes the vacation worse, not better, because I end up feeling guilty and bad. Staying in control of my eating on vacation makes the whole trip better because I feel so much better. And then I won't have to worry about getting back on track when the vacation is over because I will have been on track the whole time.

To reinforce these messages, I asked Karen to consider how she wanted to feel when she got home. First I had her imagine that she had significantly overeaten on vacation and gained weight. As she visualized herself getting on the scale the morning after she arrived home, she saw herself feeling bloated and heavy and discouraged, as indeed she had felt after last year's vacation. Then I had her imagine that she had stayed in control and had gained at most only a pound or two. Now she felt lighter, proud, encouraged, and optimistic. She wrote another card:

I want to carry the good feelings of the vacation with me when I go home. If I eat with abandon, I'll feel bloated and heavy and discouraged. But if I stay in control, I'll feel light and proud and encouraged and optimistic. It will be so worth it to stay in control.

Escape the Vegas Mind-Set Trap

We tend to look at vacation as the "no-rules zone"—but every single extra calorie you eat comes back with you as a souvenir. And when you focus on the positive consequences of sticking to your plan, you can prevent a sense of vacation deprivation.

- Make a list of the advantages and disadvantages of eating whatever you want versus the advantages and disadvantages of staying in control during your vacation.

- Recognize that eating freely while you're away doesn't feel good all the time—especially when you feel bloated or sluggish.

- If there are certain foods you have historically allowed yourself to eat only on vacation, plan to have these foods periodically throughout the year. That will minimize the special aspect of that food so you won't feel pressured to overindulge "only on vacation."

- Consider how you want to feel when you get home: happy that you stayed in control or unhappy that you've gained too much weight? Picture how much effort you'll need to expend and how much time it will take to lose your vacation weight.

- Think about your choice: to continue your cycle of vacation eating regret or to establish a new tradition that makes you proud.

#5: The Unreasonably Strict Eating Plan Trap

You make eating plans that are too difficult to follow.

Another common trap arises when you make a plan that is too restrictive. While your intentions may be good, you need to be realistic. Consider how likely it is that you will stick to your plan.

A plan that is too difficult to follow can give rise to sabotaging thoughts: "It's too hard. I'll just eat whatever I want and get back on track once I get home." But if you develop a new plan that includes extra food, you may not gain any weight at all (if you're exercising more). Or you may gain a little weight but far less than you would with an overly restrictive plan that you eventually throw out the window entirely.

When Karen and I discussed what she wanted her vacation eating plan to be, she initially said, "I guess it should be the same as when I'm home."

"Can we figure out how realistic that is?" I asked. "Didn't you say you'd be eating in restaurants most nights? And that you'd be in and out of the kitchen all day? And that you want to eat some special treats you can only get at the beach?"

Karen thought this over. "Maybe it's a good idea to be a little looser than when I'm home. Because some years, I've started off being as strict as usual, but by the second or third day I ate off plan, and then it was no holds barred. I ate out of control for the whole rest of the week."

We decided it would be a good idea to define *looser,* because Karen had already seen that being "looser" at home gets her into trouble. She recognized that looser shouldn't mean spontaneously deciding what she wanted to eat. Instead, she decided to plan extra food in advance and try to gauge how much weight she'd gain.

Karen decided that she was willing to gain two pounds at most. We also calculated that she'd probably burn some extra calories (although perhaps not a lot) by being more physically active than she is at home. She made the following plan.

Vacation Eating and Exercise Plan

Breakfast: same as home

Lunch: same as home. If I'm at a restaurant, order something that's as close as possible to something I would eat at home

Dinner: when eating at a restaurant, ½ to ¾ portion protein, ½ portion carbohydrate, one portion salad, vegetables without added butter or oil, one glass of wine, taste of dessert. Request all sauces on the side; use sparingly

Snacks: high-protein snack, twice a day

Special treats: 5 times per week, one medium-size cookie from a bakery or one small frozen yogurt or about 2 cups of boardwalk caramel corn

Exercise: 30 minutes per day, walking or bicycling

Next we discussed Karen's reentry into post-vacation life. Returning home and getting back on track had historically been a problem for her. She decided to prepare and freeze turkey meatballs before she left and to make sure that she also had frozen vegetables in the freezer, so she wouldn't be tempted to just snack and graze when she got home instead of sitting down for a proper meal. She also committed to getting on the scale the next morning *no matter what.* And for the first time, she arranged to go late to work the following day so she would have time to go to the supermarket and get the house in order for the week. She added these items to her vacation list.

I saw Karen two weeks later. She had done really well. Although she had deviated from her plan twice, she got herself back on track immediately. And she had already lost one of the two pounds she had gained. She was very happy!

Escape the Unreasonably Strict Eating Plan Trap

Dieters can be all-or-nothing about eating out, whether they're dining close to home or traveling. They frequently think they should abandon all restrictions on vacation or they should follow exactly the same plan as they do at home. Someplace in the middle is a better bet. But don't just "loosen up." Especially if you'll be away for a few days, figure out how much weight you're willing to gain, if any, and plan your food intake accordingly. It's totally reasonable—and probably important—to plan to eat a little more at meals or have extra treats. As long as you make a plan in advance and stick to it, you'll reinforce good habits, even if you do gain a pound or two.

- Whenever possible, look at restaurant menus to decide what you're going to order before eating out. If you can't, have a general plan and practice portion control.

- If you eat out often, you can't have an appetizer, soup, salad, bread, dessert, *and* wine—along with the main course—at every meal. Consider alternating the add-ons. One time add an appetizer. Another time add salad or soup.

- Most restaurants are notorious for serving huge portions. Figure out the amount of food that's comparable to what you eat at home and separate the extra food from the portion you plan to eat.

- Create a list for travel. Figure out what you need to do before you leave, while you're en route, and while you're away.

- Make sure your eating (and drinking) plan is reasonable and manageable. If you'll be away for a week or more, consider a plan that may lead to gaining a couple of pounds. That will undoubtedly be much less weight than you'd gain if you had no plan, a loose plan, or too restrictive a plan.

- If you make a mistake in your eating and get back on track right away, there will be no harm done. Watch out for a sabotaging thought about "blowing it" for the whole trip, which can give you license to eat out of control until you get home.

- Plan what you'll eat for your first meal home *before* you leave on your trip.

- Commit to getting back on the scale the morning after you get home no matter what. If you're driving to your vacation destination, you can even bring your home scale with you and weigh in daily, which will help you stay on track.

Creating Escape Plans for Travel and Eating Out

Eating in restaurants and on the road can present a variety of challenging traps. The diversity of offerings, the novelty of eating out, and a tendency to give yourself license to abandon your plan can make it difficult to stay in control. Create as many escape plans as you need to manage the different settings in which you may find yourself. Remember, every mistake is an opportunity for learning, so keep adding to these escape plans as time goes on.

❶ **Identify a future situation in which a travel and eating out trap might arise.**

❷ **Record your sabotaging thoughts.**

❸ **Write a compelling response to each sabotaging thought.**

❹ **Develop a list of strategies.**

❺ **Review and revise your escape plan often.**

Consider the following sample escape plan as you brainstorm and craft your own.

Escape Plan: Travel and Eating Out Trap

Situation #1: The brunch buffet at the hotel. I always go with good intentions of having eggs and fruit—but then I end up having one of everything.

Sabotaging Thoughts	Reminders	Strategies
This is really a special buffet and I want to get my money's worth. I may never be back here so I want to make sure to try everything. I can get back on track after this weekend. I want to be free to eat whatever I want. Everyone else will be eating whatever they want.	We've already paid for the buffet so the money is gone. It's worth a huge amount to me to stay in control so I can lose weight. I can either sample everything and strengthen my giving-in muscle or I can establish a new buffet habit, stay in control, strengthen my resistance muscle, feel good about myself, and feel physically so much better when brunch is over. How many times have I "started my diet" on a Monday? I could have lost weight and kept it off for years now, if I didn't use that excuse. I can be free to eat whatever I want or I can stop fooling myself and finally lose weight for good. Every time matters. Being free to eat whatever I want means gaining weight and feeling guilty and heavy and bloated for the rest of the day. It's not worth it. Other people may actually be limiting themselves, if they're watching their weight, following a medical diet, or restricting themselves to just the healthiest choices. In any case, what other people are eating isn't relevant to the goal I have for myself of losing weight.	Review my advantages list and this escape plan just before I go down to the buffet. Decide in advance whether to have moderate portions of eggs and fruit or small portions of several different foods. If the latter, look over the whole buffet and choose the 4 or 5 foods that look the best. Take one plate of food. When the food is gone, put my napkin on the plate to signal that I'm finished. No going back for seconds. Read reminder cards about weakening my giving-in muscle and strengthening my resistance muscle. Give myself enormous credit for staying in control. Imagine how happy I'll feel when I get on the scale Monday morning and find out I didn't gain weight!

Reflect and Recommit:
Why I Want to Escape This Trap

Consider, is it worth it to treat every meal out as a special occasion—and feel significant regret afterward? What do you need to remind yourself the next time you go out to eat? Won't overeating put a cloud over the meal? **If you get off track while you're away on vacation, won't it actually make the trip worse?**

Before you pack your bag for your next adventure or pick a restaurant for date night, set aside time to work on travel and eating out traps so you'll be prepared. Take a few minutes to write one final summary reminder card to motivate you to make changes and keep making changes.

Chapter 8

Holiday Traps

So many challenges can pop up during holidays. You might be invited to parties where other people are eating and drinking with abandon. People might bring you treats, either at the office or at home. Maybe you have a long-standing habit of overindulgence fueled by the sabotaging thought, "It's a holiday, so it's okay to let loose." You think you'll be happy if you let yourself eat freely. But is that really true? Think about the outcomes of a loss of control. Guilt, lower self-esteem, a drop in confidence, and an increase in weight will certainly put a damper on your celebrations. On the other hand, if you learn how to stay in control, you will probably enjoy the holidays much more. Prepare for common holiday traps to help you escape them.

#1: The YOLO (You Only Live Once) Trap

You use holidays as an excuse to eat whatever you want.

Staying in control at parties—especially holiday parties—is difficult for most dieters. It's so easy to get caught up in the holiday spirit and over-indulge. And while it is reasonable to plan in advance to eat a little extra, you will certainly gain weight if you go to a lot of parties during the holidays and indulge at each one.

Deanna was a secretary who worked for a telecommunications company near our office. She came to see me in late summer, in anticipation of the December holiday crunch. She told me that she was about fifteen pounds heavier than she had been a few years before, and she wanted this to be the year she turned it around. Deanna had always been a fairly consistent exerciser, and she didn't think her diet changed all that much from year to year, but there was one gigantic black hole in her otherwise effective self-care plan: the entire winter holiday season.

Deanna loved parties, and she especially loved the holidays. Until she was in her late forties, she had been able to indulge during the holidays and gain a few pounds but then lose the extra weight within a couple of months when she resumed more careful eating. In recent years, though, she was finding it harder and harder to bounce back. She would gain a few pounds during the holidays and then *not* lose it. "Every December, I promise myself I'll keep my eating under control since I obviously can't afford to do what I used to do, but then I don't. It's so much harder than the rest of the year."

Practicing the foundation strategies, Deanna lost seven pounds during the fall months. In early December, she and I agreed that it would be reasonable for her to try to maintain this weight loss until the New Year. She wouldn't focus on losing more weight until January.

Even with this reasonable goal, Deanna told me that parties would be especially challenging. "I find it so hard to really watch what I'm eating when I'm going to all these events," she said. "Being so disciplined just gets tiring and I start to lose motivation. That's when I begin to think things like, 'This is too hard. I don't want to think about this anymore. I'll just eat whatever I want for now and then I'll be really careful in January.'"

I asked Deanna what she saw as the advantages of staying on track during the holidays. We came up with a long list.

Advantages of Staying on Track During the Holidays

1. I don't naturally lose extra holiday weight anymore. If I gain weight this year, I will have to put in a major effort to lose it.

2. I'll feel more in control.

3. I won't have to worry about getting back on track in January.

4. I won't be at the mercy of cravings every time I see holiday treats.

5. I won't feel self-conscious eating in front of others at holiday parties.

6. All my clothes will continue to fit through the holidays and into the New Year.

7. I'll feel excited about holiday parties instead of feeling worried about my eating.

8. I won't worry about what to wear to holiday parties because I'll know that everything will fit and look good.

9. I'll be setting a great example for years to come.

10. I'll start the New Year in a happy place.

11. I won't undo all my good work from the rest of the year.

Deanna decided she needed to read this list regularly.

Now that it was clear in Deanna's mind why it was worth it to her to stay on track during holiday parties, we worked on sabotaging thoughts that could get in the way. "I'm not sure what to tell myself if I have the thought, 'It's the holidays. I don't want to have to think about healthy eating.'" I asked her whether *not* thinking about what she was eating had worked for her.

"No," she replied. "And now I'm convinced that I want this year to be different." She sounded determined.

"Then let's come up with a really strong response," I replied. "What do you want to say to yourself if you begin to feel tired of thinking about your eating?" Following our discussion, Deanna created a reminder card:

There's no such thing as "not thinking about" my eating. If I think about it before I go to parties (and when I'm there), I can plan to incorporate a special treat and feel really good afterward. If I don't have a plan, I'll be thinking a lot about it when the party is over—in a negative way—and I'll feel really bad that I didn't control my eating. So either way, I'll be thinking about it.

Escape the YOLO Trap

During the winter holiday season, it is so easy to undo all the work you've put into losing weight over the previous months. Some dieters loosen their control at Halloween and never really regain it until January—if at all. Others do well until the end of November, running into trouble around Thanksgiving, or December, when the round of holiday events starts. If you're working on losing weight, this season can seem like a baited trap. But if you pay attention to the foundation strategies, learn additional holiday strategies, and follow a few tips, you can get through this challenging time feeling proud of yourself *and* having fun.

- Make a holiday advantages list with all the reasons why it's worth it to you to stay on track. Read it at least once a day and before going to parties.

- Make a plan for how many treats you'll have during a holiday party *before* going to the party.

- Keep in mind that you can't take in extra calories at each party and still maintain your weight, unless you refrain from eating an equivalent number of calories during the rest of that day.

- If you're tempted to go to a holiday party and just "not think" about healthy eating, remind yourself that there's *no such thing* as not thinking about it. Either you're going to think about it now, make healthy choices, and feel good when the party is over, or you're going to think about it later—and feel bad.

- Remind yourself that it's not all or nothing. It's not a choice between eating every treat you want or not getting any treats at all. Look for the middle ground between these two extremes.

#2: The Wall-to-Wall Treats Trap

You can't avoid the holiday foods in the office kitchen.

Deanna told me that another big challenge during the holidays involved the treats in her office. "It's kind of ridiculous how much food there is at work—like baked goods in the kitchen and candy on the other secretaries' desks. Not to mention the baskets of goodies that vendors deliver almost every day." She sounded almost indignant. "It's just everywhere! I try really hard to resist, but it just gets the best of me sometimes."

I asked Deanna when it was hardest to resist. "Around three or four in the afternoon," she said. "That's when I get hungry and draggy and tired. When it's not holiday time, I just eat a piece of fruit. But there's less food in the kitchen then, of course. It's so much harder during the holidays. I frequently end up having the fruit and at least one treat."

Deanna needed a guideline for office treats. I told her about a rule I have for myself: *no junk food before dinner.*

"We frequently have treats in our office kitchen year-round, not just during the holidays, and if I didn't have this rule," I explained, "every time I went into the kitchen to get water or tea, I would see the food and struggle about whether to eat it. I'd put myself at risk for cravings throughout the day. But because I made this firm rule for myself, it really isn't difficult. It was harder to stick to the rule at the beginning, but over time, it got easier and easier because I proved to myself that I can always resist those treats. I know that if there's something I really want, I can bring some home and have it after dinner—I just can't have it at that moment. Knowing 100 percent that I'm not going to have junk food at the office makes my day *so much easier.*"

That sounded reasonable to Deanna, though she thought the rule would be really hard to stick to. "I'd like to learn how," she said. "Whenever I eat sweets at the office, I always end up feeling guilty. Sometimes I just sit at my desk and obsess about the food in the kitchen. Then I start to crave it, and eventually I give in. And then I get mad at myself."

And even worse, having one treat didn't stop the craving. Because then Deanna would *keep* thinking about the food and go back and eat more— and feel guilty again. "The cravings and gaining weight. It's just not worth it. I think I'd like to try your rule." She made the following list.

Holiday Treats

1. No to eating office treats in the office.

2. Yes to taking a piece home for after dinner—unless I have a party that night and will be eating a treat there.

3. If I have a craving, do something else (or several things) until the craving passes:
- Refocus on my work.
- Do some deep breathing.
- Drink water.
- Take a walk.
- Check my e-mail.
- Do desk aerobics.
- Talk to a coworker.

"You know," Deanna said, "I think I'd like to make a reminder card, too."

It's worth it not to eat junk food at work. I don't want to be plagued by cravings and I don't want to gain weight and I don't want to feel guilty afterward. If I see treats in the office that I want, remember: I _can_ have them, just not right now. I'll enjoy the treat so much more at home when I've planned to have it because I'll eat it guilt-free.

I told Deanna two other reasons I faithfully stick to my no-junk-food-at-the-office rule: "I know that if I did have a treat, I might not be satisfied with just one; I might want to keep on eating. Also, my confidence would go down. Giving in would make it harder in the future, because I might think, 'Well, I gave in yesterday or last week, so maybe I'll give in now, too,' as opposed to knowing *I just don't give in*. That way, I don't even have to think about it."

Deanna nodded. "I'm going to add those things to my reminder card."

Escape the Wall-to-Wall Treats Trap

You'd think that with so many people trying to resist this trap, office workers and colleagues everywhere—at least those who are trying to eat healthfully or avoid gaining weight—would simply declare a cease and desist on break-room treats! But until this idea catches on, you need to protect yourself.

- Consider making guidelines for yourself about how many office treats, if any, you're going to have. For many dieters, it works to have the rule "One treat a day and no treats while I'm at the office" or "No treats in the office except Friday after lunch."

- Remind yourself that if you make the rule "No treats at work," it's not as if you can't have the treat you want; it's just that you're not going to have it at that moment. You can take it home and enjoy it after dinner.

- Every time you stick to your rule, give yourself loads of credit.

- If you're tempted to break your rule, remind yourself that *every time matters* because every time you're strengthening either your giving-in muscle or your resistance muscle.

- Bring a healthy snack with you to work so you won't be as tempted.

- Think about how you've handled holiday treats in years past. Did you overeat? Did you gain weight? While it may be hard in the moment to resist office treats, you'll be happy you did once you leave the office for the day.

#3: The Fit-In Foodie Trap

***You tell yourself it's okay to indulge
because everyone else is doing it.***

When Deanna came back to see me the following week, she told me that though she was doing much better with the treats at the office, she had experienced a disheartening problem on Saturday afternoon.

"I was at a friend's holiday party," she told me, "and it just didn't go well. I went in with good intentions, but then we started decorating cupcakes and everyone was eating them, so I did, too, even though I had already had my treat. There were lots of other holiday foods that I didn't even touch, but I definitely shouldn't have had the cupcakes."

Deanna had decided before she went to the party that she'd have one treat. She ate several cookies soon after she arrived. "And that should have been it," she said. "But the cupcake decorating caught me by surprise. I started thinking, 'Everyone else is having one, so it's okay if I do, too.' And then, once I ate one cupcake, I thought, 'Well, other people are having another, and besides, it's holiday time.' So I had most of a second. And then my friend offered me a taste of hers. It was red velvet cake, which I had always wanted to try, so I had a few bites of it. I really blew it."

Deanna's sabotaging thoughts were typical. She needed a strong reminder card so the past wouldn't repeat itself.

What anyone else is eating is irrelevant. The fact that it's a holiday season is irrelevant. I need to focus on what I have to do to avoid gaining weight. Holiday calories are the same as all other calories. If I eat extra treats, I'll gain weight. It isn't true that it's okay to eat this because it's holiday time. It's not okay if my goal is to maintain my weight.

"One more thing about the party," I said to Deanna. "You said there was other holiday food you didn't even touch. Looking back, do you regret not eating more of the food that was there?"

"No. I'm glad I didn't eat even more."

"But you do regret eating the cupcakes?"

"Yes, definitely."

"That's really important. Most dieters get to the point where they don't end up regretting the food they *didn't* eat. They only regret the extra food that they *did* eat."

"I think I'm at that point. I feel really good all day long when I stand firm at the office, and after I had the cupcakes, I was definitely sorry."

In response to this idea, Deanna made the following reminder card:

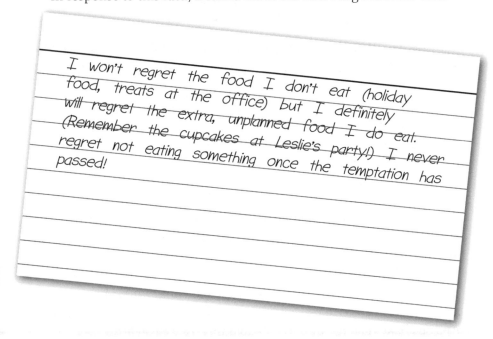

I won't regret the food I don't eat (holiday food, treats at the office) but I definitely will regret the extra, unplanned food I do eat. (Remember the cupcakes at Leslie's party!) I never regret not eating something once the temptation has passed!

Escape the Fit-In Foodie Trap

Peer pressure, herd mentality, social contagion—whatever you call it, we have to remain aware of its ability to sway our eating behavior, particularly when we're looking for an excuse to eat.

- Remember, extra calories are extra calories. The fact that other people are eating treats or that it's a holiday is irrelevant. If you don't want to gain weight, you can't take in extra calories.

- Ask yourself, when I get home from the party or get on the scale the next day, am I going to regret it if I didn't eat extra food? Or will I regret it if I did?

- When you resist temptation, give yourself lots of credit.

- After you've successfully navigated a holiday event, create a "worth-it memory" entry in your journal to celebrate your accomplishment and remind yourself the next time of your strength.

#4: The Before the Big Day Trap

You get loose with your eating even before the holiday starts.

Kathleen loved entertaining friends and her large brood at holidays. The mother of four grown children, Kathleen had nine grandchildren and two more on the way. She had been doing quite well and was gradually losing weight. At a session in early November, we began to discuss Thanksgiving.

I asked her to describe a typical Thanksgiving holiday. She told me that the entire family and some close friends descend on her home in late morning and stay the whole day. They had developed a number of rituals over the years: a pickup game of touch football (with even some of the little ones playing), looking at photographs of the family at holidays from years ago, helping Grandpa do yard work, and eating lots and lots and *lots* of food.

Around noon, Kathleen puts out pigs in a blanket, several kinds of gourmet cheeses and crackers, exotic dips and chips, stuffed mushrooms, and miniature crab cakes—all before the luncheon feast is even served! And she bakes enough dessert, she told me, "to feed an army."

I asked Kathleen how she felt last year when Thanksgiving was over. "Well, I felt okay until I looked at the photos the kids e-mailed me," she said. "Then I felt pretty bad. I couldn't believe I looked so big."

It was difficult to get her eating back under control. "I hated gaining weight and undoing all my hard work. But it's such a strong pattern with me," she said. "I start to get looser with my eating the day before Thanksgiving. I have all these foods in the house that I normally don't buy. I tend to taste everything I bake. . . . Then I eat way too much on Thanksgiving and sometimes for the next few days, too. Within a few days, I've sometimes gained back everything I had lost in the previous month!"

Kathleen needed some solid plans: one for the days leading up to the holiday, one for the holiday itself, and one for the days following the holiday. Plus she needed reminder cards to help her stick to these plans. She decided to have an "eat normally rule" for the day before Thanksgiving. This meant having roughly the same schedule for eating that she had been following, though she could plan *in advance* to incorporate some special foods into her meals and snacks. For example, she usually didn't keep nuts in the house but knew she would buy pecans to make a pecan pie. She could plan to have pecans for her afternoon snack in place of what she usually had.

The one exception to unplanned eating would be when Kathleen legitimately needed to taste some of the dishes she was cooking. She decided that would be the extent of the extra food she'd consume before the holiday itself. She started a list.

The Day Before Thanksgiving

1. Eat normally. Follow my usual schedule: breakfast, lunch, snack, dinner, snack.

2. If I want, plan in advance to substitute (don't add) special food (like pecans) into my meals and snacks.

3. No spontaneous substitutions.

4. Do only necessary tasting.

5. Read my advantages list and reminder cards as needed throughout the day.

Kathleen realized that a reminder card would be helpful, too.

If I get tempted by extra food (crackers, dips, etc.) in the house that I haven't planned in advance to eat, remind myself that I want to start a new tradition of healthy eating this year. If I want to feel good, I have to stick to my plan.

I asked Kathleen to describe what her day would look like. "I get up really early, around five o'clock, to start baking—my specialty," she said with pride. "I also make side dishes and hors d'oeuvres. I have to set the table, usually for about twenty-five people. And I always end up having to run out to the supermarket for last-minute ingredients." She sighed. "I get really tired. Then it's hard to stay in control."

"When will you be *most* tempted to stray from your plan?"

Kathleen pondered the question. "When I'm baking," she said. "Especially when I'm transferring the cookies from the cookie sheet to the serving plates, and they're all warm and smell so good. That can be my downfall." Kathleen and I discussed her options:

- Skip making the cookies altogether—and avoid that temptation.

- Make the cookies right after breakfast when she was feeling full and less likely to be tempted.

- Plan to make the cookies and not have any.

- Decide in advance to have a certain number of cookies fresh out of the oven (which she would eat sitting down, slowly and mindfully).

- Save the cookies for her evening snack so she could look forward all day to having them. A few seconds in the microwave would warm them up.

Kathleen chose the fourth option and added it to her list.

Have 2 cookies as soon as they've cooled down a bit. Eat them sitting down. Eat slowly and enjoy every bite, guilt-free. Have a piece of fruit for my evening snack instead of my usual sweets.

Escape the Before the Big Day Trap

When you get caught up in an exciting time, even the few days before a big event can feel celebratory. If you're in the kitchen more, this could be an especially vulnerable time for you.

- If your usual routine is interrupted by being a host, make a preholiday eating plan so you won't be so tempted to eat spontaneously.

- Schedule your day to include exercise and rest periods.

- Put tempting party food items in grocery bags (even the ones in the refrigerator) until just a few minutes before the guests arrive to minimize your exposure to them.

#5: The Perfectionista Trap

You spend too much time and energy making everything "just so."

With further discussion, it became apparent that Kathleen would be so busy the day before Thanksgiving that she'd have difficulty sticking to her normal eating schedule. I asked her what impact this could have on her eating.

"Well, it won't be good, I admit," Kathleen told me. "I guess I'm a perfectionist. I try to make everything perfect. So I tend to let other things slip, like exercise and healthy eating."

I suggested to Kathleen that she might need a new mind-set. "Right now it seems you have the idea that you have to do everything perfectly, even if it comes with negative consequences, like gaining weight. Is that right?"

"I never thought about it like that." She reflected on what I had said. "Yes, I guess you're right," she agreed.

"So if you want this year to produce different results, doesn't it mean that you have to do things differently? I'm wondering if it would be good to think about not cooking *everything* from scratch. If you did, it would free up some time for you to do things like sticking to regular meals, and it would free up some energy so you could focus on healthy eating."

"Well, it probably would help. But I just can't imagine buying prepared food for a holiday!"

"It doesn't have to be all or nothing, does it?" I asked. "It's not as if you have to either make everything from scratch or buy everything. Isn't there a pretty big middle ground?"

Kathleen nodded. "That's true."

"So are there some things you could buy?"

Kathleen thought about it. "Ummmm, I actually like the dips I've gotten from the farmers' market. I could get those. And they have a really good sweet potato casserole."

Next I asked Kathleen whom she could ask to bring a dish. "My sister-in-law has offered to bring hors d'oeuvres in the past, and my daughter says she can bring homemade bread. I guess I could take them up on it. But," Kathleen sighed, "the food would be different. Everyone is expecting things to be the same."

"That may be true." I paused. "On the other hand, is it possible people might *like* something different? In any case, I wonder whether it's worth it for you and maybe some others to be a little disappointed—if it means you won't have this huge disappointment when you get on the scale after the holiday is over." Kathleen agreed and made the following reminder card:

> Not only is it okay for me to not make everything from scratch, but it's important for me not to. Buying some things or asking other people to bring things will give me more time and energy. It would be nice to take it easier. And that way I can focus more on healthy eating.

Kathleen started a new list: buying dips, a sweet potato casserole, and cut-up fruit and crudités from the farmers' market, as well as asking her sister-in-law and daughter to bring hors d'oeuvres and bread. This list proved invaluable to Kathleen, not only for this Thanksgiving but also for other holidays and other years.

Escape the Perfectionista Trap

Holidays are like catnip to those who like to entertain—but they can also be the undoing of perfectionists who are trying to lose weight. Patterns are strong and traditions run deep, but remember, you can always choose and you can always change.

- Recognize that if you don't make any changes, you'll have the same outcome as always: being unhappy with yourself when the holiday is over.

- Identify ways you can be less perfectionistic, even if it means that you (or possibly others) will be a little disappointed. Anyway, isn't the main point of the holiday to be with friends and family?

- Create new holiday traditions, such as letting other people share in the preparations—which will likely help them feel more connected with the festivities and allow them to gain a satisfying sense of nurturing, just as you do.

#6: The Big Day Trap

You overeat on the holiday itself.

Hors d'oeuvres start at noon on Thanksgiving Day at Kathleen's house, and the family sits down for their big meal at one o'clock. In years past, Kathleen skipped her usual breakfast and dinner and just snacked. She was ready to try a different plan.

To eliminate snacking, Kathleen decided to start off with her normal breakfast. She wasn't sure what to do about the hors d'oeuvres, though.

"It will be hard to eat them slowly and mindfully," she said, "because I'm either running around being the hostess or having such a good time talking to people that I barely notice what I'm eating." She decided to save two of her favorite hors d'oeuvres in the kitchen and eat them as part of her Thanksgiving lunch, when she'd be sitting down and could really appreciate them. She also decided that she would take only moderate portions of food, fitting everything (including the hors d'oeuvres and bread) on one plate without heaping it high, and would definitely skip seconds. She would also have a slightly smaller than usual dinner, with one piece of her favorite dessert.

Kathleen thought it might be difficult to avoid taking seconds, so we did some problem solving and she made the following reminder card:

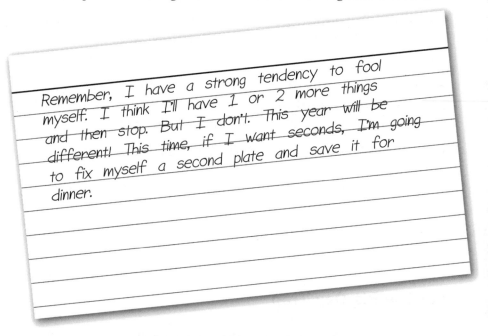

Remember, I have a strong tendency to fool myself. I think I'll have 1 or 2 more things and then stop. But I don't. This year will be different! This time, if I want seconds, I'm going to fix myself a second plate and save it for dinner.

Next I asked Kathleen whether cleaning up and putting away food would be a problem. "Yes, probably," she answered. "Usually the men and kids go outside to play touch football, and the women stand around the kitchen, talking and nibbling while we put away the food." Dealing with leftovers can be a risky proposition. Kathleen decided that she had to stick hard and fast to her "no-eating-standing-up rule." She made two more reminder cards:

During the whole holiday, I need to eat everything sitting down, slowly, and enjoy every bite, so I will feel happy when the holiday is over.

When I'm tempted to have leftovers, remind myself that this is not my last chance. I can have leftovers for dinner or over the next couple of days, so I don't need to eat them now.

"I have another idea that might help," I told Kathleen. "Do you think you'd like to start a new ritual? You and the other women could put the leftovers away as quickly as possible and then go for a walk together. That way, you won't be so tempted, and you'll get some exercise."

"I love that idea!" she exclaimed. "I'm going to do it."

Kathleen now had a robust plan for Thanksgiving Day. She made the following list.

Thanksgiving Day

1. Read my advantages list and reminder cards in the morning as usual, and at the first sign of being tempted.

2. Eat a normal breakfast.

3. Skip hors d'oeuvres but save 2 for my lunch plate.

4. Serve myself one plate of food, whatever I want, with small to moderate portions, but no seconds.

5. When I've finished, prepare a second plate of food and save it for dinner. Make it just a little smaller than my usual dinner.

6. Eat slowly and really focus on how each bite tastes so I can really enjoy it.

7. Put away leftovers quickly and take a walk.

8. Have one portion of whatever dessert I want.

Escape the Big Day Trap

Prepare for the big day in advance. Mentally review how you will handle your eating for each part of the day. Think about changes you need to make so you can feel pleased with yourself when you go to bed instead of feeling guilty or regretful about your eating. Then commit your plan to paper. Seeing it in black and white will keep you on track and accountable.

- Don't skip any meals or you'll set yourself up for overeating later.

- Eat everything slowly and mindfully, while sitting down. It's so easy to be distracted—try to get as much enjoyment as you can from every bite.

- Create a list that helps you overcome the temptation to stray from your eating plan.

- Make a leftovers rule for yourself if that has been a problem area for you in the past.

- Figure out how you can get in some exercise; invite others to join you.

- Decide when you are going to have your one serving of dessert, and enjoy every bite.

- Give yourself credit for every skill you practice and every time you stick to your plan, especially if you're tempted not to.

- Create an entry in your memory book to savor the day and remind yourself how to have a great holiday in the future.

#7: The Post-Holiday Trap

***You have trouble staying on track
when the holiday is over.***

For many, the sheer quantity and variety of leftovers after a holiday meal or party provide an overwhelming temptation. Kathleen recognized that post-Thanksgiving leftovers constituted a clear and present danger. She needed to think through her options and settle on a plan, which she recorded in a list.

Post-Holiday

Returning to normal eating will be so much easier than in past years because I will:

1. Encourage family and friends to take home leftovers (make sure I have containers and ziplock bags for them).

2. Save my leftovers in individual portions.

3. Throw away food that could be too tempting. It's not worth the struggle. Better to waste it in the trash than in my body.

When Kathleen came back to see me several days after the holiday, she told me about her experience, reporting that she had done "pretty well." Actually, she had done great! She'd stuck to her plan, except that she started to nibble on leftovers as she was cleaning up and putting food away. She realized that she had made an excuse. "It really won't matter. It's just a few tastes." But then she reminded herself that it did matter because it wasn't just the calories; it was also the unhelpful habit she was reinforcing. She then told herself that if she kept nibbling, she might decide that she had blown it and junk her plan for the rest of the day. And she knew from past experience that sometimes she didn't get back on the wagon for days afterward.

"And then what happened?" I was curious to know.

"I stopped," Kathleen said.

"How great!" I told her. "And were you proud of yourself? Did you give yourself credit?"

"Actually I did," she said. "And I was also proud of myself the next day when I stayed in control."

Kathleen told me she had been mightily tempted by the leftover cherry pie. The day before, she had wrapped the extra three slices individually and put them in the back of the refrigerator. But she saw them when she was putting away food after lunch. She rationalized that she'd have her piece of pie right then instead of waiting for after dinner, as she had planned. So she ate it. But she hadn't enjoyed it much, because she ate it too quickly and felt guilty. Feeling unsatisfied, she wanted more. But instead of getting a second piece, she put the other two pieces down the garbage disposal.

"It's the first time I ever got rid of food because I knew it would be too hard to have it around. I felt really good about it," she beamed. "I took control instead of letting the food control me."

I told Kathleen how impressed I was with how well she had done. "There were probably dozens and dozens of opportunities for you to go off plan, but you only made two mistakes—and even then you caught yourself and turned things around!" Using her new strategies, Kathleen had created a very different holiday experience. She maintained her weight and her sense of control. She told me that she felt much more confident about tackling other holidays now that she had a blueprint. She wrote an entry in her memory journal to commemorate her achievements and her sense of pride.

Escape the Post-Holiday Trap

Many dieters know they need a firm plan for the holiday itself. But they don't recognize that they may also need a strong plan for the days following the holiday, when company may still be visiting or leftover food calls their name.

- Create a good plan that will serve you well not only in the aftermath of this holiday but also for all the post-holiday days to come.

- If leftover food could be a problem, ask your guests to take leftovers home with them. Collect plastic containers and ziplock bags to have on hand before they leave.

- If you still have food around that could put you at risk for eating off plan, throw it out. You'll avoid the "should I or shouldn't I eat it?" struggle that you might otherwise end up losing.

- If you have trouble getting rid of leftovers, list the costs of throwing away food versus the costs of keeping the food.

Creating Escape Plans for Holiday Traps

Escape plans for holiday traps require a full-frontal attack, because you may have many, many temptations to contend with. Anticipate situations that may be difficult. Make sure you're prepared in advance with a plan. When you are tempted in the moment, remind yourself of how you want to feel when the holiday is over.

❶ Identify a future situation in which a holiday trap might arise.

❷ Record your sabotaging thoughts.

❸ Write a compelling response to each sabotaging thought.

❹ Develop a list of strategies.

❺ Review and revise your escape plan often.

Consider this sample escape plan as you brainstorm and craft your own.

Escape Plan: Holiday Trap

Situation #1: The entire span between Halloween and New Year's Day. I'm feeling hopeless about being able to stick to my diet.

Sabotaging Thoughts	Reminders	Strategies
There are just too many parties, too much food, too much temptation. It will be too hard to stay in control. It will be easier if I stop dieting now and start again in January. I won't have a good time if I can't eat and drink the way I want to.	It may be hard but it's certainly not impossible. This year is different from the last few years when I didn't know how to motivate myself every day, how to manage cravings, or how to answer back my sabotaging thinking. This year it's going to be easier to stay on track. Instead of thinking about the whole holiday season, just focus on one day and one party at a time and remind myself that of course I can follow my eating plan that day. I don't want a repeat of the last few years. I was so unhappy in January when my clothes didn't fit. And then it took me weeks to really get back in the saddle and another month to lose all the weight I had gained. Besides, it's not easy being overweight! That's really hard. It doesn't have to be all or nothing in terms of holiday eating. I can plan to have one special treat and one drink at every party. I may gain a pound or 2, but that's fine! And it's not as if food is the only determinant of a good time. Talking to people (and flirting!) are actually more fun.	Focus on staying in control one day at a time. Create a special holiday advantages list to read at least twice a day. Read relevant reminder cards and this escape plan twice a day. Create an image of waking up on January 2nd and feeling so good about myself because I stayed in control over the holidays. Write out what that image looks like in my notebook. Plan to have one special treat and one drink at each party. Focus on connecting and having fun with people at each party.

Reflect and Recommit:
Why I Want to Escape This Trap

Do you want to keep treating every holiday as a free-for-all—leaving you with extra holiday pounds? **Do you want holidays to continue to be a source of frustration or do you want to transform them into happy occasions?** You have the opportunity to set a new precedent with a new approach, one that will make you feel good about yourself, in control, and strong.

Commit yourself to working on your holiday traps right now, so you'll be prepared. Take a few minutes to write one final summary reminder card to motivate you to make changes and keep making changes.

PART FIVE

Universal Traps: How We All Get Trapped

Chapter 9

Psychological Traps

Just about anyone who has ever struggled with dieting has been afflicted with traps of the psyche. Most psychological traps involve feeling deprived, discouraged, unmotivated, or burdened by the demands of what it takes to consistently eat in a healthy way. These feelings are normal and fade much faster if you're prepared for them. Anticipating potential roadblocks and planning what to do will let you keep going, even when you want to abandon your efforts.

#1: The Discouragement Trap

You want to give up when dieting becomes difficult.

Chris, who worked in the insurance industry, had been coming to see me for several months. His weight problem had begun several years before, when he started a sedentary job and then injured his back—and so could no longer play basketball. He wasn't burning off calories the way he had in the past but didn't change his eating, so extra pounds started to accumulate. He had tried several times to lose weight but couldn't seem to stay on track.

Once Chris mastered the foundation strategies, began to change his eating, and started to exercise again, he lost twenty pounds fairly quickly. He was psyched. He thought losing more weight would be relatively easy.

But that was an unrealistic expectation. He didn't know that dieting gets harder for everyone from time to time, as circumstances, motivation, and energy levels change—how could it not?

When Chris subsequently had a difficult week, he became quite discouraged. He found himself struggling to stay on track and began to have a number of sabotaging thoughts, such as "I don't know if I can keep it up." When he came to see me, he said the whole week had been hard.

I asked him to take out his advantages list and read it aloud, rating each item as very important, important, or not important. I wasn't surprised that every one of them turned out to be either important or very important to him. I asked him if it was worthwhile to keep going, even though he felt discouraged, so he could get these advantages. When Chris replied yes, I asked him to make a reminder card he could refer to often, to help him keep his goals at the forefront of his mind.

> While losing weight sometimes feels difficult, the results will be worth it. The advantages on my list are too important to give up on, no matter what I may think or feel at any given time.

Something interesting happens to many dieters when they've had a hard week, and I suspected that it had happened to Chris. The memory of a few difficult hours colors their perception of the week as a whole.

I asked Chris if all 168 hours of the past week had been difficult. "Well, I was sleeping for some, so those weren't hard," he laughed.

I asked for an example of a time that was particularly hard. He described his experience at Sunday breakfast, when he had gone with friends to a diner known for its large portions. He'd been tempted to eat all the hash browns and toast on his plate.

"Did you struggle the whole time you were at the diner?"

Chris thought about it. "No, it was only when I finished what I had planned to eat and wanted more. So maybe it lasted about ten or fifteen minutes, until the waitress cleared the plates off the table. Once my plate was gone, I didn't think about it anymore."

I reviewed Chris's week with him in some detail:

"Were other breakfasts hard?"

"Nope, those weren't a problem."

"How about the periods between breakfast and lunch each day?"

"Nope."

"Lunch?"

"Nope."

"Between lunch and dinner? Dinner? After dinner?"

When Chris really thought about it, it turned out that the only other times that had been especially difficult had been about an hour midafternoon on Saturday, three dinners out with clients (but only when they were eating dessert and he wasn't), and a couple of evenings when he had finished his allotted treat but still wanted more.

All told, he calculated that only six or seven hours at most had been difficult.

When Chris realized that most hours weren't hard—and, in fact, were neutral or even easy—he felt much better. He made the following reminder card:

When I get discouraged, count up the hard hours. Remember that every hour of every day isn't difficult. In fact, there are many more easy or neutral hours than hard ones.

Then Chris shared another sabotaging thought: "I still don't know if I can keep it up for the long term, though. Even though I know all the hours last week weren't hard, the ones that *were* hard felt *really* difficult. I'm worried I'll eventually get tired of dieting and give up. That's what has always happened in the past."

But this wasn't the past. What was different about how he was going about dieting this time? We created a substantial list:

- He was only making changes in his eating that he could keep up for life—no more crash diets or unreasonable restrictions.

- He could still have his favorite foods; he hadn't eliminated bread or beer or desserts as he had in the past.

- He had learned to eat moderate portions of favorite foods and enjoy every bite.

- He had learned how to motivate himself with his advantages list.

- He had learned how to give himself credit for successes and constructively learn from challenges.

- He had learned how to plan his eating, stick to a schedule, and eliminate spontaneous eating.

- He had started to change his thinking, thanks to repeatedly reading his reminder cards.

Looking at the list, there was no doubt: this time was truly different. His previous attempts to lose weight had been much harder. He would be good for a few days, and then lose it and go completely off plan. He had really struggled. But, thinking back, he realized how different his mind-set and behavior were now. And come to think of it, though the past week had been more difficult, the preceding six weeks or so had really been okay. Chris realized he needed another reminder card for the next time he got discouraged:

> If I start to worry that I won't be able to keep going, remember that things are very different this time. I've learned how to eat in a way that I can keep up long term. I've learned how to get myself to stay on track. I've learned how to deal with hunger and cravings and how to counteract my sabotaging thoughts. Plus I've made my giving-in muscle MUCH weaker and my resistance muscle MUCH stronger.

After some additional discussion, Chris decided another reminder card would be helpful, one that got him to focus just on the present moment.

When I'm going through a difficult time and start thinking about the future, change my focus. Think about right now. Can I stay in control at this moment? If I have a problem later on, I can solve it then.

Chris also resolved to remind himself that a year from now he'd also have twelve more months of practice under his belt.

I don't have to worry about how I'll be able to stay in control in the future because by the time the future comes, I'll have had so much more practice and be so much better at staying on track. When I face tough times, I'll find it easier to say, "Big deal, so it's been hard during a few hours this week. I've gotten through lots of weeks like this. I know I can get through this one, too."

Escape the Discouragement Trap

When you've tried and failed to lose weight in the past, you sometimes drag all those negative memories into subsequent attempts. Like Chris, you may vastly overestimate just how much of the week was difficult. You may believe that you shouldn't experience difficult times when it's actually abnormal for dieters *not* to struggle from time to time. And you may even stop practicing your foundation strategies. All these factors can give rise to the unhelpful idea that you can't keep it up. So when you feel discouraged, consider doing the following:

- Take out your advantages list. How important is each item to you? Write down *very important, important,* or *not important* next to each one.

- If any advantage doesn't feel important at that moment, consider taking it off your list so you can focus on the reasons that are most meaningful to you. If you need shots of motivation during the day, read the list frequently.

- Count the difficult minutes and hours. How many hours did you struggle? How many hours *didn't* you struggle?

- Think about previous attempts at dieting. What have you learned since then? Remember that two months from now, if you keep practicing the foundation strategies, you'll be in an even better place than you are right now.

- If you feel overwhelmed, you're likely taking too long a view. Instead ask yourself, "Can I keep this up right now?" Take it one moment at a time.

#2: The Deprivation Trap

You feel resentful for having to restrict what you eat.

Catherine came into my office when she was on a break from her most recent show. A vivacious actress and dancer with a dramatic flair, Catherine traveled with a touring company that performed in different venues each week. That lifestyle had lent itself to such undisciplined eating that she'd gained nearly fifteen pounds on tour, despite the amount of exercise she was getting during rehearsals and shows. She only confronted her weight gain when her manager warned her that she needed to lose weight if she wanted to have her contract renewed. While she did lose a few pounds before coming to see me, her motivation had begun to wane, especially at dinner and in the evening.

"I smell pizza, or someone orders french fries, and I can barely resist ordering them myself," she confessed to me. "I dream about eating cake and ice cream. Food is all I think about! I know I'm eating in a healthier way than I was at the beginning of the tour, but I'm bored with it now. I can't eat *anything* I want. I'm tired of depriving myself!"

This sense of deprivation was getting in the way of Catherine's sticking to her plan—and it was also starting to threaten her career.

"I know I need to lose more weight—my manager has warned me about this enough times," she sighed. "But I just really wish I could start eating foods I like again!"

"Catherine," I asked, "do you have the idea that when you're following a healthy eating plan, you can't eat any foods you enjoy?" I asked.

"Well, I know I can have them from time to time but, on the whole, no," she said. "It's mostly just salads while everyone else is eating hamburgers and onion rings."

Two of Catherine's ideas gave me pause:

- When she was following a diet, she couldn't eat foods she enjoyed.

- She could only eat salads, while everyone else ate what they wanted.

It sounded to me as if part of the reason Catherine was feeling so deprived lately was because she actually *had* been depriving herself. She was displaying classic all-or-nothing thinking. She didn't recognize the huge middle ground between being able to eat everything you want whenever you want and not being able to eat anything that you enjoy. I asked her what she thought would happen if she continued to feel deprived. "I'll eventually end up going in the other direction and eat way too much," she said. "But if I do eat my favorite foods, doesn't that mean I'll gain weight?"

"Not at all," I explained. "When you have a reasonable plan to incorporate your favorite foods, you may slow down how quickly you lose weight. But isn't that worth it if it means you can lose weight and keep it off long term?"

Following our discussion, Catherine made the following reminder card:

If I start feeling deprived, ask myself, am I being too restrictive? It's important to incorporate my favorite foods into my diet (even if it means I lose weight more slowly) or I'll rebel, give up, and gain weight back.

Catherine then expressed concern that even if she could eat her favorite foods, she likely couldn't eat as much of them as she would like.

"There's just something so great about sitting down with a big plate of pasta or a big bowl of chili with cheese and a big hunk of corn bread, and eating it all. But I know I can't do that."

"Well, you're right," I said. "You probably can't eat all your favorite foods in large quantities and still lose weight. But let me ask you a question: What will happen if you don't lose weight?"

"I won't get my contract renewed."

"And would you be unhappy about that?"

"Yes, I love my job! That would be terrible. Like, worst-case-scenario terrible."

"Okay, so it might be helpful to keep this in mind. Either way you're going to be deprived. You'll either be deprived of some food, in some quantities, some of the time—but not all food all the time. Or you'll be deprived of *everything* on your advantages list, including keeping your job. Which would be the bigger deprivation to you?"

Catherine's eyes opened wide. "Wow, I hadn't thought of it that way. Losing my job would be *so* much worse than not being able to finish a plate of pasta." She made the following reminder card:

> I will be deprived either way. I'll either be deprived of some food some of the time (but not all food all the time), or I'll be deprived of everything on my advantages list, including my job. Which deprivation do I want?

I also wanted to address Catherine's assertion that everyone else got to eat burgers. As long as she kept telling herself that "everyone else" could eat that way, she would continue to feel deprived. But was it really accurate?

When I asked her to think about this a bit more, she realized that she had been thinking of the meals she ate with the young men in the troupe. She laughed as she realized she'd been comparing herself to men in their early twenties, whose metabolisms were clearly much faster than her own. To say "everyone" ate whatever they wanted was clearly inaccurate.

I asked her to describe to me what the women her age and older ate. "Egg-white omelets, chicken, veggie wraps, salads, things like that," she said. "Yeah, I guess they do eat less than the guys!"

"So what does that tell you?" I asked her.

"That I'm not the only one limiting my eating," she admitted. "I guess the other women are, too. I think I need a reminder card."

> I can't compare my eating to that of a young man (who's not trying to lose weight) because I'm not a young man. I need to remember that I am eating 100% normally for someone of my age and gender with my weight-loss goal.

Escape the Deprivation Trap

Have you always had the mind-set that dieting means giving up the foods you love? This is probably part of the reason you've gained weight back. This time, focus on what's reasonable for you to do long term.

- If you're feeling deprived, check to see if you're being overly restrictive. It's possible that the reason you feel deprived (or part of the reason) is because you actually *are* depriving yourself more than necessary. If so, that degree of restriction can set you up for failure.

- If you *are* being too restrictive, take steps to incorporate some favorite foods into your daily eating. While you may experience slower weight loss, you will enjoy mealtimes more and avoid feeling overly deprived. You'll be eating in a way that you can maintain long term.

- Keep in mind that there is a vast difference between eating *every* bite of food you want and eating *nothing* you want. Yes, it's true that you may need to limit the quantity or frequency of some foods. But you will either be deprived of some food some of the time (but not all food all of the time) or you'll be deprived of the life-enhancing, lifelong advantages on your advantages list. Which is the bigger deprivation?

- Remember, there's no such thing as good food and bad food, but there are foods you should eat more of and foods you should eat less of.

- Redefine your concept of "normal" eating. Catch yourself if you're comparing yourself to someone with a faster metabolic rate or someone who isn't trying to lose weight.

#3: The No Willpower Trap

You believe you can't resist overeating.

Catherine had been doing well for months, but one day she sounded quite discouraged at the beginning of our phone session. She told me about an experience she'd had a few days before at the wedding of two cast members. Things hadn't gone well.

Although she had decided beforehand to have one piece of wedding cake, her plan flew out the window once she saw the dessert tables piled high with goodies. She ended up eating several desserts and tasting even more.

"It was just too hard," she said. "There were so many desserts that looked good. I just had no willpower. I couldn't resist; it was impossible."

Catherine hadn't been overcome by circumstances. She had been overcome by sabotaging thoughts. Telling herself that she had no willpower gave her an excuse to give up trying to control her eating.

Catherine and I talked about the difference between things that are hard and things that are impossible. "It may be really *hard* to resist a craving in the moment," I explained, "but it is definitely not impossible. Walking on the ceiling, defying gravity—that's impossible. But isn't resisting a craving in a different category altogether?"

"I know what you're saying," she said. "But in the moment it felt so hard." She was right. It had been really hard. She needed to be better prepared the next time.

To build her confidence that she could overcome difficulties, I asked Catherine to tell me about some difficult things she had accomplished in her life. She told me that one of her greatest and most difficult achievements was getting cast in the current show. She had been required to go through audition after audition and endure long hours of dance instruction and rehearsals.

That was a great example. Now, what had she done in terms of dieting that had felt really hard? Well, she recalled, she had gotten her eating under control when she was on the road. She had resisted overeating tempting food on the boardwalk on her day off this past week. And come to think of it, she had turned down lots of junk food that the cast brought to rehearsals and performances—soft pretzels, saltwater taffy, chocolate-covered caramels.

I asked her to think about all these experiences. "Was it easy to exert willpower in those situations, or did some of them feel difficult?"

"No, they weren't all easy," she admitted.

"What does it tell you about your ability to do hard things?"

"I guess I can."

"You guess you can?"

I could tell from her voice that she was smiling. "I know I can."

I suggested that Catherine capture some of these triumphs in her memory journal. "And when you got through those situations without giving in, how did you feel afterward?" I asked Catherine. "Did you regret sticking to your plan?"

"No, not at all. Not ever. I always felt great. And proud of myself."

Catherine made the following reminder card for these important ideas:

> There is a difference between things that are hard and things that are impossible. Just because it feels really hard to resist eating something, that doesn't mean I can't. I have done many other hard things in my life and have resisted many hard cravings. It's not always easy, but it _always_ feels fantastic and worth it.

Escape the No Willpower Trap

It's always possible to exert willpower in any situation because eating is never automatic. Giving in is always a result of being overwhelmed by sabotaging thinking—not because a situation is truly unmanageable. Being prepared and having a plan greatly increases the likelihood you'll be able to exert willpower in even the most difficult situations.

- Check to see what kind of language you're using with yourself. If you tell yourself some food is "impossible to resist" or you have "no willpower," remind yourself that these phrases just provide an excuse to indulge. Keep in mind the difference between things that are hard (or really hard) and things that are truly impossible.

- Make a list of the hard things you've done in your life—raise children, get a degree, work toward a promotion, learn a sport. All those endeavors took sustained effort and determination. They were hard, but you did them. Next make a list of difficult dieting experiences in which you stayed in control. Remember that even though it's hard, you can exert willpower and resist—and when you do, you won't regret it once the tempting situation has passed.

#4: The Feeling Overburdened Trap

You get tired of focusing on and putting effort into weight loss.

Linda has been overweight almost her entire life. When she first came to see me, she weighed just under three hundred pounds. Her weight was greatly affecting her life and her health. She was prediabetic, had high blood pressure, and was on a host of medications to help with health problems that, as her doctor kept telling her, her excess weight was greatly exacerbating. Linda also cared for her elderly mother, who had difficulty getting around. Both of them had mobility issues.

As Linda and I worked through the initial skills, she felt very committed and did well. She dutifully worked on her foundation strategies every day.

The first few months, Linda was thrilled with her steady weight loss. She still had a long way to go, but she felt in control of her eating for the first time she could remember. However, a few months into treatment, her mother injured her arm, and Linda suddenly found herself having to do much more for her mother than she was used to.

"I have so much to think about right now," she told me. "Things with my mother are really difficult, and I have to say I'm just tired of having to think about my eating. I'm tired of having to make healthy choices all the time, and I'm tired of having to put in all this work."

Many people who are trying to lose weight eventually get to this point: feeling burdened by having to work on healthy eating. They usually have sabotaging thoughts along the lines of "I'm tired of having to work on this" or "I just don't want to have to think about it right now."

I told Linda how sorry I was that things felt so difficult for her. I could certainly understand how the process of losing weight might feel like one more gigantic burden that she didn't want to think about. But here was the truth: she would be burdened either way. I asked her to consider some other burdens she was carrying right now. How burdensome was it for her, at her current weight, to

- help her mother around the house?

- go up and down the stairs?

- spend time worrying and feeling bad about her weight?

- go to doctors' appointments?

- deal with the cost and side effects of medications—all due to the extra weight she was carrying around?

We agreed that dieting is also burdensome. Of course it is. It requires a fair amount of time and energy and thought. But at least you get a great payoff. Linda made the following reminder card:

Either way I'm burdened. Either I'm burdened by having to work on healthy eating, or I'm burdened by being overweight (physically, mentally, emotionally, and financially). At least when I work on healthy eating, I get so many positive benefits as a result.

With these ideas firmly in mind, Linda was able to keep on track. "I'm so grateful that I didn't give up," she told me the following week. "Even though it's been hard at times, losing weight is absolutely worth it."

Escape the Feeling Overburdened Trap

There's no denying it: losing weight takes a big investment of time and energy. Sometimes it can feel overwhelming. But focusing on what you'll get out of weight loss—as opposed to how hard it is—will help you through tough times.

- Write down all the ways your extra weight is burdening you. Think about how it affects your health, your physical abilities, your thinking, your mood, your feelings about yourself, and your self-confidence.

- Remind yourself that either way you're burdened. Either you're burdened by everything that comes with being overweight or you're burdened by having to work on healthy eating.

- Recognize that staying overweight (which will be a constant burden in your life) comes with really negative consequences, while focusing on weight loss (which is only an intermittent burden) brings welcome consequences.

#5: The I Don't Care Trap

Momentary feelings of apathy sap your motivation.

I'd been working with Kayla, a research assistant at a local university, for a couple of months when she told me she'd been having trouble that week getting herself to practice her foundation strategies. She just couldn't seem to summon the energy. "I don't know," she said. "I felt so motivated until a few days ago. I don't know what happened."

Kayla had gotten off track a few days before. She overslept and didn't read her advantages list or reminder cards in the morning, and she skipped breakfast. She was starved by lunchtime and ate a whole burrito and chips much too quickly. A few hours after lunch, she got more chips from the vending machine down the hall—even though there was an apple at her desk she had planned to eat. "Then I guess I just gave up," she shrugged. "I ate way too much for the rest of the day." The following day unfolded much the same way.

"Okay," I said. "You overslept. Did you forget to read your cards, or did some sabotaging thought get in the way?"

"I truly just forgot to read them," she said. "And then I forgot to put them in my purse to read at work."

In this case, Kayla and I agreed that forgetting her cards was just a practical problem. She just needed to make an extra copy of her advantages list and reminder cards to keep in her purse. But lunch was when things had gotten difficult.

"Did you forget to eat slowly and mindfully? Or did you have sabotaging thinking?" I asked.

"I didn't really forget," she admitted. "I thought, 'I'm so hungry. I know I should eat slowly, but I don't care.'" Aha! She had just identified a key sabotaging thought. She continued to think, "I don't care," when she ate the chips, and then many times during the next few days.

"Now that the situation has passed and you overate, do you still not care?" I asked.

"No, I do care," she said ruefully.

"Why?"

"Because I really want to lose weight!" she said emphatically. "And because I know overeating really sets me back. Not only did I eat too many calories, but I know I've been strengthening my giving-in muscle."

Kayla clearly cared an awful lot after the fact. This would be important for her to keep in mind in the future: her moments of not caring are fleeting and temporary, and she *always* cares later because losing weight is really important to her. Kayla made the following reminder card:

The next time I think, "I'm going to eat this because I don't care," remind myself that while it's true I may not care right in that moment, I absolutely will care later on—so I can't let this one moment of not caring dictate my actions.

When dieters have the thought, "I don't care," it is momentarily true. Or is it? I encouraged Kayla to remember the exact moment when she stood in front of the vending machine.

"You said that you got chips instead of eating your apple because you were thinking, 'I know I shouldn't get these chips, but I just don't care.'"

"Right," she confirmed.

"Think back to that moment. Which do you think you wanted more in that moment—to lose weight or to eat the chips?"

"In that moment, I really felt like I wanted the chips. I just didn't care. I wanted those chips, and I was going to eat them."

"Okay, let's play a little game," I said. "Let's say that right when you were standing in front of the vending machine, the Instant Gratification Genie appeared to you and said that you could instantly lose weight or eat the chips. Which would you choose?" Of course Kayla chose losing weight. "So what does that tell you about your thought that, in the moment, you just didn't care about losing weight?" I asked.

"I guess I really did. If I hadn't, I would have taken the chips, no matter what."

Kayla made the following reminder card:

Even when I tell myself I don't care about losing weight, I really do. There's never a time when I wouldn't choose to lose weight over anything I was about to eat.

Escape the I Don't Care Trap

The lure of food can be powerful. Sometimes we just don't feel like exerting the energy it takes to stay on track. That's when we pretend to ourselves that we don't care about the consequences of going off plan. But obviously we really do care.

- Think about all the times you gave in to the I Don't Care trap. How did you feel after the fact? How do you feel now?

- Keep in mind that the "not caring" feeling *always* passes, but the reasons you want to lose weight will not stop feeling important.

- Recognize that while it may be true that you don't care in the moment, it's not true that you won't care later on. But also question whether you *actually* don't care at any given moment. If the Instant Gratification Genie appeared to you in those moments, would you choose losing weight? Or would you choose the food?

Creating Escape Plans for Psychological Traps

The psychological traps in this chapter plague just about every dieter. It's normal to feel discouraged, burdened, deprived, unmotivated, or apathetic from time to time. To avoid being blindsided by these temporary negative states of mind, prepare yourself by creating your own escape plans.

❶ **Identify a future situation in which a psychological trap might arise.**

❷ **Record your sabotaging thoughts.**

❸ **Write a compelling response to each sabotaging thought.**

❹ **Develop a list of strategies.**

❺ **Review and revise your escape plan often.**

Consider this sample escape plan as you create your own.

Escape Plan: Psychological Trap

Situation #1: I feel so discouraged. It just feels like this whole week was so hard.

Sabotaging Thoughts	Reminders	Strategies
The whole week was hard.	Actually, the whole week wasn't hard. It was hard for about 7 hours. Dieting is supposed to get hard from time to time. It gets harder for everyone. Remember how hard it used to be? It's easier today than it was a year ago. And it will be a lot easier a year from today as long as I keep practicing my skills and don't give up.	Write down how important every advantage on my advantages list is to me.
It shouldn't be this hard.		Read my advantages list 3 times throughout the day.
I can't keep it up.		
I wasn't able to keep it up in the past.		Count up how many hours were actually difficult this week and how many hours weren't.
It's not worth it to keep it up.		
Even if I keep it up for now, I won't be able to keep going in the future.	I'm just making an excuse because I don't feel like making the effort right now. I can, in fact, keep it up this moment.	List the foundation strategies I have already learned.
	Now I know how to diet. I didn't know how before.	Give myself double credit for staying on task when it feels difficult.
	It is worth it, to get the advantages on my list.	
	Although I should expect some hard times in the future, dieting will get easier and easier the more I practice my skills. A few months from now, my skills and my resistance muscle will be stronger than they are today.	Read over my "worth-it memories" to remember how wonderful it feels when I stick to my plan.

Turn my attention to right now. I can certainly keep it up for today. |

Reflect and Recommit:
Why I Want to Escape This Trap

You have a choice: you can keep allowing these psychological issues to get in the way or you can use the strategies in this chapter to address sabotaging thoughts.

- If you feel discouraged, think about all the easier hours of the week and focus on just doing what you need to do today.

- If you feel deprived, think about which deprivation you'd rather live with—being deprived of some food or being deprived of *all* the benefits of weight loss?

- If you feel burdened, ask yourself which burden you want: the burden of controlling your eating (but just think of the payoff!) or the many burdens of being overweight?

- If you feel a lack of willpower, remember how you were able to persevere in the past when you had an important goal.

- If you feel apathetic, remind yourself that you will very soon care greatly if you give in and overeat.

Working on psychological traps will help you plow through the difficult times and keep your motivation steady. Take a few minutes to write one final summary reminder card to help motivate you to make changes now and in the future.

Chapter 10

Getting Off Track Traps

Almost every dieter who has had trouble losing weight or maintaining a weight loss has had a specific kind of sabotaging thought after eating off plan, something like this: "I've blown it. I might as well give up, eat whatever I want for the rest of the day, and start again tomorrow."

But just think: What if, every single time in the past you had made a mistake with your eating, you had immediately recovered and gotten right back on track? What if you had automatically said to yourself, "Oh, no big deal," and continued to eat in a normal controlled way? Wouldn't you be much better off now?

Making a mistake can derail you for a day, a week, or even a year, but it doesn't have to. Once you learn to see a mistake in eating as just that—a mistake and not a license to eat wholly out of control—it will become much easier to get right back on track.

You probably have a different view of making mistakes in other areas. Think about any new undertaking you've pursued—maybe a sport, a hobby, or a new challenge at work. Did you expect yourself to be instantly perfect? Did you become demoralized and immediately quit when you made one mistake? Making mistakes is truly part of the learning process. We hope you said to yourself, "Oh, well, I made a mistake. That's to be expected. Just let me find out how to do it right." And you kept going.

But what happens when you make a mistake in dieting? If you're like most chronic dieters, you are probably extremely hard on yourself. You chastise yourself; you may label yourself as lazy or weak. Even after a single unplanned cookie, you might tell yourself, "Well, I screwed up—might as well give up for today." This sabotaging thought ensures that you will keep making one eating mistake after another. Instead, you need to learn how to immediately regroup, carefully assess why the mistake happened, and decide what you can say and do differently next time.

The *initial* dieting mistake is not the real trap here. The trap is what happens *afterward*.

#1: The I've Blown It Trap

You tell yourself you will get back on track tomorrow.

Jeffrey never had a problem with his weight until he hit his midthirties, when he got married and started leading a more sedentary life. Now he was much heavier than he had been a decade before, despite many attempts to lose weight. He always did well for a few weeks or even months. But then "something" inevitably happened, and he got off track, felt demoralized, and abandoned his weight-loss efforts altogether.

Jeffrey described a typical problematic situation. A few months earlier, when he was once again trying to curb his eating, he was watching football at a buddy's house. There was a big assortment of food, and he was tempted by the pizza and wings. He soon ate too much. Once he had "broken" his diet, he just kept overeating, telling himself, "I've blown it for the day. I might as well keep eating and start again tomorrow."

Did he go back on his diet the next day? He laughed ruefully. "No, I didn't. I was kind of on-again, off-again for a while. I kept promising myself every day that I'd be 'good,' but it took a long time to really get back in control." Jeffrey told me how discouraged and disappointed he had been with himself day after day after day.

What's interesting about this kind of "blown it" thought is that in almost no other area of life do we think it makes sense to compound one mistake with another. Consider these "mistake analogies" and notice how irrational they sound. Let's say you were walking down a flight of stairs and stumbled down a few. Would you think, "I've really blown it now!" and throw yourself down the rest? Or imagine you were driving on the highway and missed your exit. Would you think, "Well, I've blown it now!" and drive five more hours in the wrong direction? Of course not. You'd immediately change what you were doing to avoid further negative consequences. When Jeffrey thought about his mistakes this way, he was able to see how illogical it was to keep making mistakes in dieting. He made a reminder card:

> When I make a dieting mistake, remember that it makes no sense to keep making more. Just as I would never consider throwing myself down any more stairs if I stumbled, I shouldn't consider continuing to eat off track.

When you learn to stop yourself after a first mistake, you put yourself in a better position than if you stop after two mistakes. And obviously two mistakes are better than three, because each time you make a subsequent mistake, you're strengthening your giving-in muscle that much more. And calories do keep adding up. Every extra mistake contributes further to weight gain.

This concept made sense to Jeffrey. "I guess I've been buying into the idea that the damage has already been done so I might as well keep eating," he said. "When I was watching the game that day, it would have been much better if I had limited my mistake to just one extra piece of pizza."

"Right! Or if you put a more positive spin on it, you've made a mistake, but you can save yourself so many calories—and start strengthening your resistance muscle— the moment you catch yourself and stop."

Jeffrey made the following reminder card:

There's <u>no such thing</u> as blowing it for the day. Every bite of food I continue to eat has extra calories. The more calories I eat, the more weight I gain. Getting back on track at any point puts me in a better position than if I wait even one moment longer.

You can work hard to prevent mistakes, but you can't eliminate them altogether. Mistakes happen. They're part of life—and they are *certainly* part of dieting. Once you make a mistake, you can blame yourself and become demoralized. Or you can *learn* from your mistake to avoid making the same one in the future.

The "three-question technique" can help. Whenever you make a mistake, take a few moments and ask yourself:

❶ **What was the situation? What happened?**

❷ **What sabotaging thoughts did I have?**

❸ **What can I say and/or do differently next time?**

Then make reminder cards based on your answers to the third question.

Here's how Jeffrey responded to these questions in relation to a second occasion (a party at his neighbor's house) when he had gone off track.

❶ **What was the situation? What happened?**
I was having such a good time. There was lots of good food there that really tempted me. I didn't have a plan going in for how much I should eat, so I ended up overeating cheese and crackers, chips and dip, and cookies.

❷ **What sabotaging thoughts did I have?**

This food looks really good. It's okay to eat it because everyone else is eating it.

❸ **What can I say and/or do differently next time?**

- *I need a plan before I go. Not having a plan never works.*
- *My body doesn't know or care what everyone around me is eating. No matter what, if I overeat, I'll gain weight.*

When Jeffrey came to see me the following week, he told me about his Sunday afternoon. He had been watching football at a bar with some friends. "I had a plan going in, but I was distracted by the game. I found myself starting to overeat, and that old thought came to mind—the 'I've blown it' idea," he told me. "But then I remembered the visual of throwing myself down more stairs, and I was able to pull back. I stopped eating. In fact, I didn't eat anything else for the rest of the game."

Jeffrey felt proud that he was able to get back in control. He knew if he had kept eating, he would have felt overstuffed, sick, and mad at himself. But because he got back on track, he was able to enjoy the rest of the game, and the rest of that day, without feeling guilty about what he was eating. "I definitely *walked* down the rest of those stairs," he told me.

Escape the I've Blown It Trap

We have found that people who never had a weight problem and never struggled to lose weight just accept eating mistakes. "I wish I hadn't eaten all those chips and dip. Oh, well, it's over and done with," they might say. And that is the end of it. No recriminations, no subsequent uncontrolled eating. In fact, they might naturally eat a little less for the rest of the day, without thinking much about it, because they just aren't hungry. They keep eating mistakes in perspective.

That's the mind-set you need to adopt so you don't fall prey to sabotaging thinking that leads you to make mistake after mistake.

- Remind yourself that in almost no other area of life would you think it made sense to compound one mistake with another.

- Write a few additional "mistake analogies" of your own. (Start with these for inspiration: If you mistakenly broke one plate, would you open up the china closet and smash the whole set? If you were making a three-egg omelet and dropped one egg, would you throw the rest of the eggs on the ground?) Visualize the one that resonates most strongly.

- Keep in mind that there's no such thing as "blowing it for the *day*," because every bite of food you eat means your body taking in more calories and gaining more weight. It all matters, and it all adds up!

- Catch yourself at the first mistake. Immediately read your advantages list and relevant reminder cards to get yourself back on track right away.

- Use the three-question technique whenever you make a mistake so you'll be better equipped for the next time. Create a list or a reminder card to avoid making the same mistake again.

#2: The Self-Criticizer Trap

You beat yourself up about making a mistake.

One of the youngest agents in her real-estate firm, Marisa describes herself as a "go-getter." She has always been hard working, high achieving, and hard on herself. Marisa grew up in an accomplished family that set strict standards for performance and behavior, which led her to work hard and shine in her career. However, it had also taken a toll on her. "I feel terrible about myself," she told me at our first appointment. "I'm thirty-two, and I'm about sixty pounds overweight." Marisa constantly beat herself up about her weight. "It's so frustrating," she said, "I'm able to be so disciplined in the rest of my life, but I just keep failing at dieting."

I knew what Marisa didn't know: the reason that she hadn't yet been successful at losing weight and keeping it off was because she didn't know how. Marisa hadn't considered that she didn't have the information she needed to be successful because, I suspected, she thought dieting should be a no-brainer. If she just worked hard at it, she should be successful, just as she was in her career.

"When you were studying for your real-estate license," I asked her,

"Did you just show up for the test? Or did you take a course and study? Did you learn how to price houses and how to figure out the risks and benefits in certain kinds of deals—or was all of that intuitive?"

"I had to study pretty hard," she said. "I took courses and learned a lot about mortgages and deeds and laws, and I shadowed three other realtors at the agency. I had to sit for the licensing exam. I really did a lot of work."

"And if you hadn't done those things?" I asked.

"Well, I would have failed, of course."

Losing weight also entails learning, but this was a difficult notion for Marisa to fully buy into. Like many dieters, she didn't think there was anything to learn. She just had to eat less. As a result, she berated herself every time she ate something she wasn't supposed to. "Like yesterday," she said. "I ate too much at a business lunch. Afterward I just felt so weak. Disgusted with myself."

"So once you make a mistake," I said to Marisa, "and you start beating yourself up, what happens to your mood?"

"I feel worse."

"And once your mood is worse, does it make it easier or harder to get back on track?"

"Way harder," she said, sighing heavily. "That's what happened yesterday."

The fact of the matter is that once you make a mistake, the worst thing you can do is reprimand yourself. The only outcomes of self-criticism are to demoralize you further, decrease your self-confidence, and make it *less* likely that you'll immediately get yourself back in control. If you share Marisa's unrelenting standard, "I should be perfect on my diet," mistakes can feel pretty painful. But mistakes are an inevitable part of any learning process.

I asked Marisa to recall when she learned to play tennis, her favorite sport. Did she make any mistakes? "Oh, I made a lot of mistakes at first," she said. "I hit a lot of balls into the net or out of bounds." When I asked her how she improved at the game, she said she kept taking lessons and practicing. "What do you think would have happened if every time you made a mistake, you beat yourself up and told yourself how terrible it was?"

"I would have felt horrible. I probably would have given up."

"But you didn't give up," I responded. "So what was your expectation about learning to play tennis?"

"I knew I wouldn't be very good at the beginning, but I would get better. And I have. Of course I still make mistakes, just not as many."

I smiled. This was the *exact* attitude she needed to have about dieting.

As long as you have the unhelpful and impossible rule "I shouldn't ever make dieting mistakes," you'll continue to criticize yourself, feel terrible, and be at risk for giving up. But there's no need to! Just as Marisa had practiced and gotten better and better at getting the ball over the net, she could get better and better at dieting, as long as she kept "taking lessons" and practicing. And she needed to recognize that, without a doubt, she *would* make mistakes along the way, errors that she didn't deserve to criticize herself for. To help her hold on to this idea, Marisa made a reminder card:

> Learning to diet is like learning to play tennis. I'll make mistakes, but that's part of the learning process. As long as I keep my expectations reasonable and keep practicing, I'll get better and better at it. Beating myself up just gets in the way every time.

When Marisa came back to see me the following week, she told me that although the reminder card was helpful, she did fall into the old pattern of criticizing herself when she ate more than she had planned at dinner two evenings before.

"I just felt so weak and stupid," she told me. "And I haven't been able to get myself back in control since. It's been such a bad week." She felt terrible. Her confidence had taken a big hit.

I knew Marisa tended to be self-critical and all-or-nothing about mistakes, so I figured it was highly likely she'd actually done better than she remembered. If she had focused excessively on her errors, she would probably have a distorted perception of the week as a whole.

I questioned Marisa carefully to find out if, even though she had made some mistakes over the past week, she had still managed to do some things well. I asked her:

- "Did you eat breakfast sitting down, slowly and mindfully, on any day?"

- "Did you eat lunch sitting down, slowly and mindfully, on any day?"

- "How about dinner and snacks?"

- "Did you overcome any cravings?"

- "Were there any times when you were tempted to eat when you were stressed or bored but didn't?"

- "Did you read your advantages list or reminder cards?"

Through this detailed questioning, a very different picture of Marisa's week emerged. She realized that she had practiced many of her dieting skills. But she had paid attention only to her mistakes and had failed to give herself credit for all the ways she was succeeding.

"One or two mistakes in no way negate all the great things you do in a day," I told her. "What do you think would happen if you started paying more attention to all the things you're doing well?"

"I guess I'd have a more balanced picture. Maybe I wouldn't criticize myself as much." She thought for a moment. "You're right. I probably did focus too much on my mistakes. But it's really hard not to!"

"What if your best friend came to you and said, 'I can't believe I left my phone at home. It has my calendar for the day on it. I can't believe I did that. I'm so weak and stupid for letting that happen.' What would you say to her?"

"I would tell her that's ridiculous. She's human. She has to expect to make mistakes. Maybe she needs a better reminder system. And I'd point out to her all the hundreds and hundreds of times she hadn't forgotten her phone."

"Exactly!" I said. And maybe Marisa needed a better reminder system, too. She thought the following reminder card would help:

If I feel like I'm having a bad week, ask myself, is that an accurate picture of what's going on? What am I still doing well? Remember that a few mistakes don't cancel out all the positives.

And Marisa decided, at least for the time being, to have a message pop up on her smartphone three times a day:

I may make a mistake today, and if I do, it doesn't mean I'm weak or hopeless. I wouldn't think that about Jamie if she made a mistake.

Practicing these new ideas, Marisa was finally able to start giving herself credit for practicing her skills and engaging in positive eating behaviors. Over time, she became less self-critical not only about eating mistakes but also about mistakes in other parts of her life.

Escape the Self-Criticizer Trap

Self-criticism plays no beneficial role when you're dieting. It just leads to discouragement and undermines your confidence. And self-criticism is usually unwarranted, the result of unreasonable standards.

- Consider this: When you were learning to play an instrument or a sport, did you make mistakes? Where would you be if you beat yourself up every time you did?

- Banish the word *cheat* from your vocabulary, at least in terms of eating. "Cheating" on your diet implies you did something morally bad. You didn't! You just made a mistake.

- Watch out for "shoulds": "My eating should be perfect." "I should never make a mistake." Rules like these ultimately set you up for failure because they're impossible to achieve.

- Remember it's not a question of *if* you'll make a mistake, it's *when*. Accept your imperfection and move on. Turn your attention to something else.

- Make a list of the foundation strategies you've still practiced, even when you feel like it's been a bad week. Pay particular attention to giving yourself credit.

- Be sure that you're taking an accurate look at what is going on and that you're not overly focusing on what you think you did poorly.

- Remember that if you wouldn't beat up your friends for making a mistake, you shouldn't beat yourself up for making a mistake. You're human, just as they are.

#3: The Overcompensation Trap

You make a mistake and decide you won't eat anything else for the rest of the day.

Brianna, an office assistant and part-time student, struggled with this trap. She attended brunch at a friend's house one Saturday and couldn't believe how much food was served. She ate "way too much." When she left the brunch, she felt guilty.

I asked Brianna what had happened next. "Well," she said, "I got home around three. I figured since I had eaten so much, I shouldn't eat anything else that day to make up for it. But I guess around seven o'clock, I started to get really hungry. I ended up ordering Chinese food and ate a huge amount. It was really bad."

Perhaps you've had this experience, too. You overeat and then decide to eat little, if anything, for the rest of the day. But at some point you get hungry. If you've promised yourself you're going to make up for your mistakes in an overly restrictive way, you get a little anxious and think, "It's too hard to deal with this hunger. I've already overeaten today, so what the heck." If you do, you may very well wind up eating much more food than if you had just decided to eat normally, or close to normally, for the rest of the day.

Deciding not to eat anything is a punishment. When you make a mistake, you don't deserve punishment. Not to mention that fasting doesn't work; you usually overeat again later in the day. It's better to modify your eating to some degree rather than to plan to eat nothing.

I discussed this more forgiving—and more practical—strategy with Brianna. We agreed that skipping her afternoon snack and having a slightly smaller than normal dinner would have been more reasonable. She decided to implement this plan if she found herself in a similar situation in the future.

"But what about when I make a smaller mistake," she asked. "Like having my treat earlier in the day instead of waiting until the evening?" After some discussion, Brianna decided in that circumstance, she would forgo her usual evening treat and substitute a piece of fruit. "That way I wouldn't be punishing myself because it would just mean that I'd already had the treat."

Brianna made the following reminder card:

> When I make a mistake, don't plan not to eat.
> It just doesn't work. I don't deserve punishment.
> It was only a mistake.

Then she created a list.

If I Overeat

1. If I make a small mistake, eat normally for the rest of the day.

2. If I have my evening treat in the afternoon, substitute a piece of fruit in the evening.

3. If I make a moderate mistake, like I did at Jane's brunch, skip my afternoon snack but eat a normal dinner.

4. If I make a big mistake, skip my snack and have a somewhat smaller dinner.

Escape the Overcompensation Trap

Look at your dieting history. Do you try to fast or severely limit your food intake after you've overeaten? How well has that worked? If it hasn't consistently worked well for you, it's time to make a change.

- Create an overeating list. Do not err on the side of overly restricting yourself (remember, it doesn't work!). If you've already eaten a significant amount, you can decide to eat a smaller than normal dinner or forgo your usual dessert that night.

- Watch out for sabotaging thoughts that can interfere with implementing your new plan. Make reminder cards to respond to thoughts like "I overate. That's bad. I'm not going to let myself eat anything for the rest of the day" or "Since I've already messed up, I might as well keep eating and get back on track tomorrow."

#4: The Stuck Off-Track Trap

You have a tough time restarting your diet after you've gotten off track.

About two months after starting our work together, Brianna went away for ten days. She canceled the appointment we had made for her first week back and didn't reschedule for another two weeks. When she did return, I could tell she was discouraged. She explained to me that she had gotten off track during her trip and had been unable to regain control.

"It just feels so hard right now," she told me. "Even if I got on track, it seems like it would take such a monumental effort to *stay* on track."

I asked her to recall her experience at a family reunion she had attended the week before her trip. "What was your eating like that day?"

"It was really good," she recalled. "I made a plan and stuck to it." I asked her how difficult it had felt to do that. "It was pretty easy. But I can't imagine being able to do that now."

Then I asked Brianna to think about how difficult it had been in the weeks before the reunion. She recalled that for the most part, it hadn't been difficult to stay in control. "I had a good groove going," she explained.

My point exactly.

Struggling to get back on track is *much harder* than *being* on track, because once you build up positive momentum, dieting gets easier. If you're like most yo-yo dieters, when you stop following your plan, you get mired in the struggle it takes to start up again. And something interesting probably happens to your memories and your thinking. You begin to believe that dieting has *always* been a struggle and always will be. You lose confidence in yourself. You forget how much easier it was when you were consistently following your plan, and you don't realize that it will get easier again once you're back on track.

"You're right. Where you are right now is really hard," I told Brianna. "And if it were always this hard, then maybe trying to lose weight wouldn't actually be worth it. But fortunately, this difficulty you're having now? It's temporary. And once you get back on track, it will get easier." Brianna made the following reminder card:

> Remember, getting back on track is hard, but that's only temporary. Once I'm back on track, things will feel much easier again.

I asked Brianna to contrast how she had felt before the reunion with how she had been feeling the last few weeks. "I've been feeling pretty crummy," she acknowledged. "When I'm off track, it tends to color my day. I feel bad about myself."

Then Brianna identified an important sabotaging thought. "It's funny," she reflected. "When I'm off track, I always think I'll be happier if I can eat whatever I want. But then when I do, like I have these last three weeks, it really doesn't feel good at all." She wanted to remember that.

Even though it's hard to get back on track, it's 100% worth it because being off track and feeling out of control feels crummy. Eating out of control actually doesn't feel good. Being on track and staying in control feels so much better.

Brianna told me she was still worried. Even though she felt committed to getting back on track, she was afraid she'd continue to make mistakes and get thrown off again. I asked her to remember the staff lunch she had attended a few weeks before she left for her trip. She recalled that overall she had done well, though she did have an unplanned pastry. "But then I just skipped dessert after dinner."

"So you made a mistake," I summarized, "and got right back on track and stayed on track. And didn't something similar happen the week before at your friend's house? What does that tell you about making mistakes?"

Brianna realized that she had made mistakes when she was on track in the past. She hadn't been perfect, but the difference was that every time she did make a mistake, she recovered right away. Brianna wanted to remember that, too, so she made another reminder card:

I've made mistakes even when I was on track, but I got right back on my plan. When I had coffee at Mathew's. Rob's retirement dinner. The staff lunch. Aunt Cindy's birthday. So I know I can do it. And I know I'll be very glad I did.

Then we came up with a specific plan to get Brianna firmly back in control. Since she was having trouble practicing all the foundation skills at once, we decided she should practice just a few initial skills to rebuild her confidence. Once she remastered those skills, we would add more back in. She wouldn't follow a specific eating plan this week. She'd just be careful about portion sizes.

Brianna created a list.

Restarting

1. Read my advantages list and reminder cards every day.
2. Eat everything sitting down, slowly and mindfully.
3. Give myself credit.
4. Watch portion sizes this week (but don't count calories).

When Brianna came back to see me the following week, a very different person entered my office. She told me that her week had gone very well. Focusing on just a few strategies boosted her confidence and left her feeling much more in control. As the weeks progressed, Brianna and I added back in every skill that she had learned before she left for her trip, and soon she was fully back on track.

Escape the Stuck Off-Track Trap

Remember that struggling to get back on track is much harder than actually being on track. Once you have built up positive momentum, dieting gets much easier. Try to keep this longer-range vision in mind when you're feeling stuck.

- Recall experiences when you stayed on track even though the circumstances were difficult. You have the skills to get yourself on track and to stay on track; you just have to tap into them.

- Think about how much better you feel when you're on track. In fact, when you're on track, you don't even question whether dieting is worth it. Being off track and feeling out of control are really hard and feel terrible. It's worth it to get back on track.

- If you feel demoralized, remind yourself that the situation isn't hopeless. Create a list of strategies and reminder cards for the sabotaging thoughts that have been getting in your way.

- If you've gotten significantly off track, start practicing just the first few foundation strategies for a week, remaster them, and regain confidence that you can do them consistently. Then gradually add in the more difficult skills. Before you know it, you'll be practicing them all again. Take it step by step.

#5: The All-or-Nothing Trap

Once you eat something "bad," you tell yourself you're "totally off track."

When Jeffrey, whom you met at the beginning of this chapter, came to session one day, he told me that the week had started off really well, but he "lost" it on Thursday. "We were out for dinner. I was really hungry, and even though I knew I should have had something like chicken, my brother ordered lasagna and I decided to have that, too. It was a really big portion, but I ended up finishing it. Then I had tiramisu and then more dessert when I got home. I was totally off track." Jeffrey clearly had a lot of all-or-nothing thinking about his eating. He viewed himself as either "completely on track" or "completely off track."

And what happened when he told himself he was completely off track? "Well, the more I say that, the more I guess I use it as an excuse to eat whatever I want," he confessed.

We talked about a middle ground: Was it possible to make a mistake, like eating too much dinner and dessert, and yet not be totally off track? Jeffrey recalled his cousin's engagement party. "I hadn't planned to have cake at lunch but I did have a slice. But then I got right back on track for the rest of the day." Jeffrey made the following reminder card:

> If I catch myself thinking, "I'm totally off track," remember that this is just an excuse. I can get right back on track immediately, like I did at Will's party. I'm never "totally off track" because being on track is always just one eating decision away.

"Next," I said, "can we talk about this idea of 'good' foods and 'bad' foods? What do you think would have happened if you truly believed it was okay to have lasagna? Maybe not a restaurant-size portion but a reasonable-size piece? Would you then have said, 'I'm off track so I might as well have tiramisu?'"

"No," Jeffrey said, "I don't think I would have."

If you really like foods such as lasagna, you're not going to be able to eliminate them forever, and you shouldn't! You just need to learn to eat moderate portions and really enjoy them. You'll still lose weight. Maybe not as quickly as you'd like, but having categories of "good" and "bad" foods is unhelpful. For Jeffrey, eating only "good" foods and cutting out "bad" foods had not helped him lose weight; he'd actually *gained* weight following this policy.

Next Jeffrey and I made a list of his "bad" foods and planned when he was going to have a moderate portion of some of them in the coming week. We also discussed the importance of his eating them without guilt. Jeffrey made the following list.

Planning to Eat Favorite Foods

1. Stop labeling some foods as bad.
2. This week, have a moderate portion of one favorite food every day.
   Monday: One beer while watching the game
   Tuesday: Half portion of french fries (plus hearty salad) at
      fast-food restaurant
   Wednesday: Single-serving bag of chips at lunch
   Thursday: A candy bar
   Friday: Two beers at McCloskey's
   Saturday: One beer and half portion of pasta at restaurant
   Sunday: One ice cream treat

Then Jeffrey made himself a couple of reminder cards:

It has never worked for me to have "good" foods and "bad" foods, because whenever I eat a "bad" food, I give myself permission to keep eating off track. And telling myself I'm totally off track leads to eating more and more "bad" foods and _staying_ off track.

There's no food I can eat when I'm off track that I can't also eat when I'm on track. And when I eat it on track, I enjoy it much more because I don't feel guilty about eating it.

The following week went considerably better for Jeffrey. He was still having a little trouble wrapping his mind around the idea that he didn't have to eliminate certain foods, but after a few more weeks of practice, he became more confident about this way of eating. He needed to have lots of experiences to fully grasp that it was beneficial to plan to have his favorite foods, because doing so actually helped him stay on track and lose weight.

Escape the All-or-Nothing Trap

Do you look at food and eating in black-and-white terms? An all-or-nothing orientation can give rise to all kinds of difficulties. A flexible approach, in which you don't totally eliminate any food you enjoy, will get you much farther.

- Ask yourself if you have a good food / bad food mentality. If so, make a list of all your "bad" foods—but label them "favorite" foods. Keep adding to the list as you think of others. Plan to have one of these foods, in a moderate portion, every day this week. If you're eating one of these foods at home, buy or prepare just a single serving to eliminate the temptation to eat more than one portion.

- Remember that there is no such thing as being totally off track. As long as you think, "I'm totally off track," you will feel out of control and give yourself an excuse for staying off track.

- If you have the thought, "It's okay to eat this food because I'm already off track," remind yourself that there is no food you can eat when you're off track that you can't also eat when you're on track. And when you eat it in an on-track, controlled way, you'll enjoy it more because you won't feel guilty about eating it.

Creating Escape Plans for Getting Off Track Traps

Unrealistic expectations, all-or-nothing thinking, harsh self-criticism, loss of confidence, a tendency to compound one eating mistake with more, and overcompensation for mistakes are common problems. Fortunately, there are solutions for all of them. What you need are escape plans to help you immediately get back on track. Remember, whenever you make a mistake, you have a golden opportunity for learning, so keep adding to your escape plans as time goes on.

❶ **Identify a future situation in which a getting off track trap might arise.**

❷ **Record your sabotaging thoughts.**

❸ **Write a compelling response to each sabotaging thought.**

❹ **Develop a list of strategies.**

❺ **Review and revise your escape plan often.**

Consider the following sample escape plan as you brainstorm and craft your own.

Escape Plan: Getting Off Track Trap

Situation #1: Beating myself up when I make a mistake and then trying to overcompensate (which never works).

Sabotaging Thoughts	Reminders	Strategies
I can't believe I cheated. I'm so weak. I can't let myself eat anything else for the rest of the day. I'll never be able to lose weight. Maybe I should just give up.	I didn't do anything morally bad. I just made some eating mistakes. Mistakes don't mean I have a weakness in my character. They have nothing to do with weakness. All it means is that I'm human and I have to keep practicing my skills so I can handle tempting food situations better in the future. I don't beat myself up for making mistakes in using the computer or playing bridge—and I shouldn't beat myself up for eating mistakes. Fasting for the rest of the day would be counterproductive, as it always is. I don't deserve to punish myself. Making mistakes is a normal part of dieting. Every successful dieter and maintainer has made mistakes. I need to just say "big deal" and move on. If I give up, I won't get all the advantages of weight loss. The reasons I want to lose weight are so important to me. I need to just keep going.	Stop using the words "cheat" and "weak." Think about the times when I made a mistake but got right back on track and was so glad I did. Write a list of all the things I did today that I deserve credit for so I can keep my eating mistakes in perspective. Practice self-compassion. Think about what I'd say to Jessie if she made an eating mistake—then say that to myself. Don't use mistakes as an excuse to make more mistakes. Eat a little less for the rest of the day but don't fast. Think about how glad I'll be later if I get firmly back on track now. Think about how unhappy I'll be if I stay off track.

Reflect and Recommit: Why I Want to Escape This Trap

Making an initial eating mistake doesn't have to be a problem. Eating an unplanned piece of cake may not even show up on the scale tomorrow morning. But compounding the initial mistake with more—well, those compounded mistakes will show up the very next day.

If you had always known how to get back on track immediately after one mistake, wouldn't you have spared yourself years of struggle?

Work on identifying your getting off track traps right now so you'll be prepared to spot them immediately next time. Left unaddressed, these traps have the potential to turn a minor stumble into a long, prolonged fall. But if you master these traps, you can minimize the damage of all other traps. Take a few minutes to write one final summary reminder card to motivate you to make changes and keep making changes, so you can avoid or escape from your traps.

Stay Free of Traps—for Life

Now that you've read about how to tackle the traps that prevent you from losing weight and keeping it off, do you feel empowered? Ready to dig in? We hope that the stories and suggestions in these pages have given you a new outlook and that you feel inspired to adopt the skills and strategies in this book. We've taken pains to be honest; we know that many weight-loss programs make outlandish promises about how easy dieting according to their plan will be. We *know* that making lasting changes in your eating can be challenging. We know that there's no such thing as a quick fix or a magic solution. But we've seen, time and again, that our research-based, common-sense approach works, both in the short run *and in the long run.*

We also hope you see that you're not alone in your struggles! Everyone who has had difficulty losing weight or maintaining weight loss has encountered similar struggles.

Using Escape Plans for Life's Varied Traps

To leave you with a bit of extra inspiration, we want to tell you how some of our dieters have used the skills they learned to escape from their traps to make meaningful and significant changes in other aspects of their lives.

Do you remember Maxine from the family trap? She had to conquer sabotaging thoughts about asking her family to make changes at home. When she came back to see me for a routine "booster" session a year after our treatment ended, I asked her which parts of our work together had been particularly helpful. Maxine told me that she had finally learned to be assertive with her family—and that had made all the difference.

Maxine had learned to stick up for herself, telling her husband that she wouldn't be eating a second dinner with him when he came home at nine o'clock because she had already eaten with the kids. She then introduced more changes into the household. Maxine told me she had had an "Aha!" moment when I asked her, "Why is it okay if *you're* unhappy, but it's not okay if Mike is unhappy?" That question had been a turning point for her. She began to recognize that she had been acting unentitled in other ways. She began to grasp, for the first time in her adult life, that her needs and desires were as legitimate as everyone else's.

Not only had Maxine instituted changes around food, meal preparation, and eating, but she also gradually started asking the children (and to a lesser degree, her husband) to help more around the house. She got the kids to do dishes, make their beds and straighten their rooms, put away their clean clothes, and pack their backpacks. These and other changes she made in running the household freed up time for her to exercise more often, visit with friends, and read for pleasure. She really felt her new mind-set had improved her life—and actually benefited her family in giving more responsibility to the children.

"For the first time, I truly began to feel like it was okay to take care of myself," she told me, her eyes lighting up. Maxine had dropped forty-seven pounds altogether, and she looked younger and more energetic. She talked about a trip she and Mike were taking that was two weeks away. "I'm going to wear a bathing suit—and even though I'm not a beauty queen, I'm not going to worry about it!" she announced proudly. "I love to swim, and I haven't done it in years!"

You also may recall Marisa, whom you met in the chapter on getting off track. Marisa drove herself very hard and criticized herself harshly whenever she strayed from her eating plan. Then, feeling distressed, she had a hard time getting her eating under control again. I hadn't seen Marisa for several years when she scheduled an appointment.

Marisa walked in beaming. "Do you remember? You helped me lose forty pounds, and I felt so much better! Much more self-confident!" It must have shown, because soon after she lost weight, Marisa met Brian. They married a year later—"and now we have Alexis." She smiled as she showed me a picture of her eighteen-month-old daughter.

"I gained almost forty pounds when I got pregnant, which was fine," she continued. "I lost a lot of it in the first five months after Alexis was born. But I've stalled since then. I'm not beating myself up about it— which is huge for me—but I'd like to lose a little more." Combining motherhood with her job had made following her original eating plan a challenge. "My eating has gotten a little sloppy. That's why I'm back. I think I just need a tune-up to get completely back on track."

First Marisa and I discussed whether it was reasonable for her to lose the additional weight. "I think so," she told me. "I've been grabbing some meals, and I know they're just too high calorie. And I'm eating too quickly, so I don't feel satisfied and then I overeat."

I reminded Marisa of something I had told her at our last session together. It doesn't work for many people who have gotten off track to focus on changing what they're eating right away. They need to do what they had done initially: master the foundation strategies one by one and just be careful about their eating until they get to strategy #9, adopt an eating plan.

Marisa and I developed a plan for her to begin practicing her foundation strategies again. We needed to problem-solve around issues of time so Marisa would be able to practice her skills, including eating slowly while sitting down and enjoying every bite. Although she wouldn't follow a specific food plan for a few weeks, we discussed how she could free up time to make sure she always had healthy food to eat at home and in the office. Marisa was optimistic that she would succeed. I told Marisa how delighted I was that her life had taken such a positive turn.

Then I asked her whether there had been any other spin-offs from our work together. She said there had been. "Before I came to see you," she explained, "I was a big perfectionist. In fact, that's why I always had trouble getting back on track. Whenever I made an eating mistake, I used to think, 'Well, I've blown it. I'm so weak. I've failed again.' And then I'd give up, for the day or the week or sometimes even a few months. But you helped me see that I had ridiculously high standards in dieting."

"Then I looked around and I realized that I had ridiculously high standards in other areas, too." I asked Marisa for an example. "Well," she said, "now that I'm working three days a week instead of five and a half, I just can't get as much done. I think I would have been really stressed out by that a few years ago. But now I'm okay with it. And I'm much more relaxed about things at home, too. Which is good, because things can get really messy when there's a baby around. Life is so much less stressful when you allow yourself to be human!"

Chris, whom you met in the psychological traps chapter, often got discouraged with losing weight, especially when the going got tough, because he expected that dieting should always be easy. He didn't have confidence that he could get himself to do hard things, and he greatly overestimated just how difficult his week had been. A few challenging hours colored his memory of the whole week. He learned to count the difficult hours, reassess the importance of each advantage of losing weight, remind himself of what he had been learning, and rein in his focus to whether he could keep going right now. About a year after we had finished working together, Chris changed jobs, from working in the claims department to sales. He said he had wanted to do that for quite a while, but he was always concerned that he wouldn't be able to keep motivated. He made the decision to apply to the training program after realizing that the motivational skills he had learned from our work together would be applicable to a sales position.

"When I got accepted to the training program, I wrote a list of all the advantages of working hard to get through the program. Whenever I started to have sabotaging thoughts about whether I'd be successful, I read the reminder cards I had made. Then once I started actually doing sales, I made a new card to read before every sales call to remind myself that I might not be able to close every sale but I needed to give myself credit for making the call anyway."

Chris also used his skills whenever he got discouraged. He reminded himself why it was worth it to keep going. And he narrowed his focus. He recognized that of course he could keep going that day. He got himself to stop looking too far into the future. "I'm pretty sure I could never have gone into sales," he concluded, "or never have been as successful as I am, if I hadn't learned those dieting skills." I laughed when he told me I should write a book for salesmen.

Chris wanted me to know one more thing. "This was really big for me. When I started doing sales, I started smoking more. About six months later, I set a quit date, which I had done a few times in the past, but this time was different. I realized that lots of the skills I used to control my eating applied to quitting smoking." He recalled that his advantages list, reminder cards, giving himself credit, the concept of strengthening his resistance muscle, distraction, and accepting the discomfort of cravings had been particularly helpful.

Chris had tried to quit several times a few years before, "but for one reason or another, I always went back to smoking. It's been about four years now, and I'm confident I'll never smoke again. I think recognizing that I can do hard things like tolerating cravings has really been key. So thank you, on all counts." Chris, like many of our dieters, found the skills he had learned to motivate himself, handle discouragement, accept discomfort, and develop self-confidence could be transferred to taking on new challenges and persevering when working toward goals that are personally meaningful and important.

When Deanna first came to see me, she had particular difficulty with holiday traps. She wanted to be able to eat and drink freely on holidays and didn't want to think about healthy eating. As we worked together, she realized that though she tried to push away the thoughts that made her feel guilty for overindulging, she wasn't entirely successful. Plus she certainly thought about her eating mistakes when the holiday was over— and felt bad, especially when she saw how much weight she had gained and found her clothes were too tight. She learned that trying not to think about her eating didn't really work.

When Deanna finished our program, she was nine pounds lighter. She went on to lose another six pounds on her own. I ran into her in the lobby of our office building a couple of years later. She looked great. She told me she hadn't had much trouble keeping her weight down. "I've become a healthy eater. Not even holidays throw me off anymore. I weigh myself every day, and every time the scale goes up by two or three pounds, I watch what I eat more carefully and it always comes right off. It's so wonderful not to have to worry anymore about getting off track with my eating or my weight."

I asked Deanna whether anything in particular stood out for her about our work together. "Do you remember how I used to try not to think about dieting, especially around holiday time? You helped me see that of course I was still thinking about it, and it affected my mood. Well, I looked around one day and realized that I had a habit of trying not to think about things I had to do but didn't feel like doing. Like making a budget and sticking to it or keeping the house neat. I realized that pushing these things out of my mind didn't feel good in the long run. It made me feel a little out of control.

"I actually used some of the dieting skills, like creating an advantages list, for doing these things and reminding myself that I'd feel better if I didn't put things off. And that I had to establish a habit of not making exceptions when there were things I had to do. There was one reminder card that was really helpful: 'Do it anyway.' It became my mantra.

"Anyway, it's just much easier for me to get myself to do things now. My life feels more under control. I think learning the self-discipline to practice dieting skills carried over to other parts of my life. My house is in order, and I now put away a decent amount of money every month into a rainy-day fund and my retirement account. I'm just more disciplined in a lot of ways. And I just generally feel so much better."

Emotional eating had been Beth's downfall. When she first came to see me, she had a demanding job as a social worker. When she came home each night from a difficult day working with clients in crisis, she wanted to soothe herself with food. Initially, she learned to engage in distracting activities instead of eating off schedule or off plan. But by the end of treatment, she was able to accept the mild discomfort of not eating something she wanted and just turn her attention elsewhere without deliberate distraction.

She came to see me five years later. She told me that she came back because she'd gained weight. "I'm up almost ten pounds from a year ago. I've really struggled to get in control, but I'm having a hard time."

I told Beth how glad I was that she had made an appointment to see me. "I just want you to know that I give you a lot of credit for coming in. We find dieters sometimes just need a little extra help to get back on track."

"Well," she sighed, "I know what happened. I'm back to eating to comfort myself. I'm at a new agency now, in an administrative position. I have a lot more responsibility. I don't deal directly with clients in crisis as much, but I have to deal with personnel and budget problems, and things like that. I'm pretty good at keeping my eating under control during the day and on weekends, but dinner and evenings are really a problem."

Beth told me a little more about her stress-filled days and what happened when she left work. I told her I thought we should plan to have a few sessions. First, I wanted to go back to basics, starting by making a new advantages list, giving herself credit, reading her reminder cards, and eating slowly and mindfully. After that, we would work out a plan for when and what she would eat in the evenings.

I asked Beth whether her sense of over-responsibility had surfaced again. "Do you remember how we talked about this unrealistic expectation you had to solve all your clients' problems? Could some of your desire to comfort yourself have to do with expecting yourself to immediately fix all the agency's problems? On the way home every night, are you anxious about work? If you are, no wonder you want to calm down by eating."

It was as if a lightbulb had gone off in Beth's head. "Yes, I think that's it exactly." She paused. "You know what was really helpful before? When you suggested I ask myself on the way home, 'Did I do a reasonable job in helping so-and-so today?' The answer was always yes, given what I had control over and what I didn't. I think I should write a new reminder card with that question on it: 'Did I do a reasonable job today, given what I have control over and what I don't?'"

Beth returned for four more sessions. By then, she was back in control of her nighttime eating, she was feeling less stressed at work, and her weight had started to drop. "I'm so glad I came back for a few booster sessions. If the scale ever starts to go up again," she said, "I'll come see you much sooner. I don't know why I waited so long!"

Miranda, the single mother with two boys, had been stressed by her busy schedule and her rules about having to be a 110 percent mom. She still calls me about once a year, just to check in and say hello. She sounded so happy on our last phone call. She had gained a little weight back, she told me, "but that's because I'm dating again! My eating hasn't been out of control. I just decided that I wanted to be able to go out with Barry for drinks and dinner. And make him home-cooked meals he likes. They're healthy but they're more substantial than I used to eat. So I've plateaued at about five pounds heavier than when I last saw you."

"That's terrific!" I said. "I'm so happy for you. And it's great that you made a conscious decision to eat more now that your circumstances are different."

Miranda has really changed since the first day I met her. She's confident about herself, she's proud of how well her boys are doing, and she has a wonderful new man in her life. She and Barry do lots of athletic things together, sometimes with the boys and sometimes not. They go on nature hikes and ride bikes, and they kayak in the summer. She doesn't have to worry about her weight affecting her activities. Her boys are also at a healthy weight, which is even more important to her. Her older son now says he wants to be a chef because he so enjoys doing food prep with his mom.

"I am just so grateful for everything you taught me," she said at the end of our phone call. "My life has gotten so much better."

Now let's talk about you.

If you haven't already done so, now is a great time to go back to chapter 2 and start learning the foundation strategies, one at a time. As you practice your skills daily, you will strengthen your habit of self-discipline. You'll become increasingly confident that you can get yourself to do what you need to do, even when you don't feel like it.

Once you've mastered the first six skills and your self-discipline and self-confidence are strong, you can start to focus on when you eat, and then what you eat. To be honest, you could probably get by for a time without mastering those first foundation strategies. You have doubtless lost weight before without using them. *But if you use your old methods, will you be able to sustain those results?* If you want a different outcome this time—if you want to escape your personal traps for good—you need to operate differently.

Once you master the foundation strategies, start tackling the real-life problems that could throw you off track. Anticipate which traps might ensnare you (the quiz starting on page 19 can help) and review strategies to create the escape plans you will need. Don't forget that some challenging situations in your life may contain elements from several traps. For example, if you're going to visit family for a week, it may be useful to reread sections on family problems, food pushers, travel and eating out, and getting off track.

The more you practice the foundation strategies and implement your escape plans, the easier dieting and maintenance will become. But you should expect to go through periods in which losing weight or keeping weight off is harder. Don't despair! Just go back to the fundamentals and make sure you're practicing the foundation strategies. Like the dieters in this chapter, if you've stopped using your skills, don't try to institute all the changes you need at once. Start with a few foundation strategies, master them again, and go from there.

As you've seen from the experiences of dieters in this chapter, you can apply many of the skills in this book to other goals that are important to you. Do you want to enhance your work life? Home life? Health? Finances? Improve your family relationships? Strengthen your friendships or cultivate new friends? How about exploring your creative or intellectual or spiritual side? Might you have a goal to enrich your leisure time or to contribute to your community or to society?

What has gotten in the way of achieving these goals up to now? Just as your diet traps locked you into negative eating patterns, similar traps may be keeping you from pursuing or achieving other goals. Think about a specific goal you'd like to set for yourself—for example, sticking to a budget. Have you had sabotaging thoughts? ("I have no self-control. If there's something I want, I just impulsively buy it.") Do you need to develop new skills? (Maybe you don't know how to budget.) Are psychological issues (such as a sense of deprivation or lack of willpower) creating obstacles? Think about the skills that you've learned in this book. Here are just a few foundation strategies that could be applicable to a wide variety of challenges and goals:

Writing an advantages list for achieving your goal

Developing consistent behavioral habits

Composing and reading reminder cards for sabotaging thinking

Creating lists and scheduling what you're going to do when

Giving yourself credit for each step you take

Accepting discomfort

Strengthening your resistance muscle

In addition, you've read about many other strategies that are applicable to other realms of struggle and achievement:

Consulting friends, family members, coworkers, or mentors

Changing unreasonable rules, such as perfectionism and over-responsibility

Developing a sense of entitlement to make changes

Being assertive with others

Staying on track when times are difficult

We hope you'll refer back to this book whenever you need it. We also hope that you feel inspired to continue your weight-loss journey and that you feel equipped to prevent or escape from your traps. We wrote this book because we recognized that people benefit from hearing the stories of how successful dieters solved problems, learned new ways of thinking, and practiced certain key skills over and over. Once our dieters master the skills they need, they continue working on their own, and many continue to lose weight for a long time to come, but we strongly encourage them to schedule periodic "booster" sessions with us to make sure they're still doing what they need to do. In the same way, we encourage you to read through this book every few months to get your own "booster" sessions. Traps and solutions that aren't particularly relevant to you right now may take on significance down the road.

Our real hope is that once you achieve success in weight loss, you'll be inspired to go much farther, to examine your life and—with your new-found skills and greater self-confidence—to dream about all the ways you can take control and make your life better. Set goals! Figure out a plan! Use what you've learned to create a better future. And when you do, be sure to acknowledge your achievements. You absolutely deserve to feel proud of yourself and your hard work.

Onward!

Connect with Us

We'd like to stay connected so we can help you on your journey – as well as celebrate your success! We hope you'll join the conversation and become part of the Beck Diet Solution community at www.beckdietsolution.com. You'll find many additional free resources, including our newsletter and daily diet tips, videos and printable templates. You can set up consultations or diet-coaching sessions in person or by phone or Skype – or attend a workshop for dieters or for professionals who work with dieters. You can also connect with us through

Facebook: www.facebook.com/BeckDietSolution

Twitter: @thebeckdiet

YouTube: https://www.youtube.com/user/beckdietsolution

Google+: https://plus.google.com/u/0/106253759201375142724/

Finally, you can e-mail us at dietprogram@beckinstitute.org and tell us about your experience using this approach: your successes, your difficulties, your questions, your suggestions. We try to respond personally to each message, and we always learn from your stories.

We've found that staying connected to each other can help all of us stay connected to our goals. Hope to hear from you soon – good luck on your journey!

Template for Escape Plan

Escape Plan: _____ **Trap**

Situation #___ _____

_____

Sabotaging Thoughts	Reminders	Strategies

Acknowledgments

We are thankful to so many people for their talent, skill, and support. Without the invaluable guidance and input from our agent, Stephanie Tade, this book would never have gotten beyond the ideas in our heads. We are grateful to Gideon Weil and Mariska van Aalst for all their editorial assistance. We are also indebted to the wonderful staff at the Beck Institute for all their hard work, and to our families for their unflagging support.

Finally, as always, we thank the dieters, both those with whom we've worked directly and those who have contacted us with feedback. We learn so much from you and are continually inspired by your hard work and dedication to the challenging task of maintaining a healthy weight. We hope that this book helps to make that journey easier.

Notes

1. "Lose Weight Your Way," *Consumer Reports* (Feb. 2013): 26–29.

2. C. M. Grilo, R. M. Masheb, G. T. Wilson, R. Gueorguieva, and M. A. White, "Cognitive-Behavioral Therapy, Behavioral Weight Loss, and Sequential Treatment for Obese Patients with Binge-Eating Disorder: A Randomized Controlled Trial," *Journal of Consulting and Clinical Psychology* 79, no. 5 (Oct. 2011): 675–85, doi: 10.1037/a0025049, PubMed PMID: 21859185, PubMed Central PMCID: PMC3258572.

3. D. E. Linden, "Brain Imaging and Psychotherapy: Methodological Considerations and Practical Implications," *European Archives of Psychiatry and Clinical Neuroscience* 258, no. 55 (Nov. 2008): 71–75, doi: 10.1007/s00406-008-5023-1, Review, PubMed PMID: 18985299; A. B. Konova, S. J. Moeller, and R. Z. Goldstein, "Common and Distinct Neural Targets of Treatment: Changing Brain Function in Substance Addiction," *Neuroscience and Biobehavioral Reviews* 37, no. 10 (Dec. 2013): 2806–17, doi: 10.1016/j.neubiorev.2013.10.002, Epub 2013 Oct 16, PubMed PMID: 24140399, PubMed Central PMCID: PMC3859814.

4. W. Hofmann, M. Luhmann, R. R. Fisher, K. D. Vohs, and R. F. Baumeister, "Yes, but Are They Happy? Effects of Trait Self-Control on Affective Well-Being and Life Satisfaction," *Journal of Personality* 82, no. 4 (Aug. 2014): 265–77, doi: 10.1111/jopy.12050.

5. F. M. Sacks, G. A. Bray, V. J. Carey, S. R. Smith, D. H. Tim, S. D. Anton, K. McManus, C. M. Champagne, L. M. Bishop, N. Laranjo, M. S. Leboff, J. C. Rood, L. de Jonge, F. L. Greenway, C. M. Loria, E. Obarzanek, and D. A. Williamson, "Comparison of Weight-Loss Diets with Different Compositions of Fat, Protein, and Carbohydrates," *New England Journal of Medicine* 360, no. 9 (Feb. 2009): 859–73, doi: 10.1056/NEJMoa0804748, PubMed PMID: 19246357, PubMed Central PMCID: PMC2763382.

Index

ABOUT THE AUTHORS

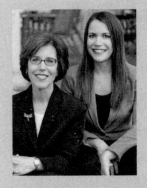

Judith S. Beck PhD is the President of the Beck Institute for Cognitive Behavior Therapy and the clinical associate professor of psychology in psychiatry at the University of Pennsylvania. Judith Beck is the author of numerous books, including the *New York Times* bestselling title *The Beck Diet Solution*.

Deborah Beck Busis is Beck Institute's Diet Program Coordinator. She works on a variety of different projects at the Beck Institute, including conducting research studies and developing a training programme and manual for diet coaches.

www.beckinstitute.org